Navigating Life
with Dementia

T0073661

Lisa M. Shulman, MD

Editor-in-Chief, *Brain & Life*® Books Series
Fellow of the American Academy of Neurology
Professor of Neurology
The Eugenia Brin Professor in Parkinson's Disease and Movement Disorders
The Rosalyn Newman Distinguished Scholar in Parkinson's Disease
Director, University of Maryland Parkinson's Disease and Movement
Disorders Center
University of Maryland School of Medicine
Baltimore, MD

Other Titles in the *Brain & Life*˚ Books Series

Navigating Life with a Brain Tumor
Lynne P. Taylor, MD, FAAN; Alyx B. Porter Umphrey, MD; and Diane
Richard

Navigating the Complexities of Stroke
Louis R. Caplan, MD, FAAN

Navigating Life with Multiple Sclerosis
Kathleen Costello, MS, ANP- BC, MSCN; Ben W. Thrower, MD; and Barbara
S. Giesser, MD

Navigating Life with Epilepsy
David C. Spencer, MD, FAAN

Navigating Life with Amyotrophic Lateral Sclerosis
Mark B. Bromberg, MD, PhD, FAAN, and Diane Banks Bromberg, JD

Navigating Life with Migraine and Other Headaches
William B. Young, MD, FAAN, FANA, FAHS and Stephen D. Silberstein,
MD, FAHS, FAAN, FACP

Navigating Life with Chronic Pain
Robert A. Lavin, MD, MS, Sara Clayton, PhD, and Lindsay Zilliox, MD

Navigating Life with Dementia

James M. Noble, MD, MS, CPH, FAAN

Associate Professor of Neurology
Department of Neurology
The Taub Institute for Research on Alzheimer's Disease and the
Aging Brain and the G.H. Sergievsky Center
Columbia University Irving Medical Center

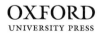

OXFORD
UNIVERSITY PRESS

Oxford University Press is a department of the University of Oxford. It furthers
the University's objective of excellence in research, scholarship, and education
by publishing worldwide. Oxford is a registered trade mark of Oxford University
Press in the UK and certain other countries.

Published in the United States of America by Oxford University Press
198 Madison Avenue, New York, NY 10016, United States of America.

© Oxford University Press 2022

American Academy of Neurology 2022

Library of Congress Cataloging-in-Publication Data
Names: M. Noble, James, author.
Title: Navigating life with dementia / James M. Noble.
Description: New York, NY : Oxford University Press, [2022] |
Series: Brain and life books | Includes bibliographical references and index. |
Identifiers: LCCN 2021057301 (print) | LCCN 2021057302 (ebook) |
ISBN 9780190495688 (paperback) | ISBN 9780190495701 (epub) |
ISBN 9780197628683 (oso)
Subjects: LCSH: Dementia—Patients. | Dementia—Patients—Rehabilitation.
Classification: LCC RC521 .M56 2022 (print) | LCC RC521 (ebook) |
DDC 616.8/31—dc23/eng/20211123
LC record available at https://lccn.loc.gov/2021057301
LC ebook record available at https://lccn.loc.gov/2021057302

DOI: 10.1093/oso/9780190495688.001.0001

5 7 9 8 6 4

Printed by LSC Communications, United States of America

"I have, so to speak, lost myself."
Translation of the case records of Auguste Deter, 1901, the first patient
described by Dr. Alois Alzheimer

CONTENTS

PREFACE

After years of training to become a specialist, all physicians, myself included, still constantly learn from our patients. We see the practice of medicine in action and learn incrementally more, patient by patient, about responses to treatment, new ideas for care, and available resources. This clinical knowledge is paired with a broader understanding of what is going on in the immense field of research. Yet for all the time spent in my practice at Columbia University Irving Medical Center—sometimes seeing a dozen patients and families in a single afternoon, every one impacted by dementia—there is never enough time for me to tell them all what they need to know and expect or to talk about all the possible challenges lying ahead. Millions of other families are also affected by dementia; some may not get the advice they need or may seek it only once critical problems have emerged.

I often lament that the practical advice my colleagues and I offer stays within the four walls of our clinical offices. I also realize that despite my best efforts to explain what we know about dementia and other neurologic problems, only a fraction of what is said may be remembered. No doubt, talking about dementia in an office visit can be overwhelming in many ways. Coming to terms with the disease, let alone understanding it, takes time. There is just so much information, instruction, and planning for care to talk about during each visit, and what we need to talk about changes from visit to visit. Despite our best efforts, we can't ever fully capture everything in notes or formal instructions handed out after a visit.

Seeing these challenges firsthand every week, I began thinking about ways to share my advice in practice with more people who need it. Once I learned of the American Academy of Neurology's Brain & Life® Books series, I was inspired to provide a "navigating" tool for people trying to understand and live with dementia. Each section and chapter of this book represents a discussion I often have with my patients and families, although it's hard to cover everything I have written about here in person, even over years of successive visits. By turning my recurring conversations into this book, I hope to help not just those seeing me in the office but also the many more families seeking answers to complex questions about dementia they may have trouble answering.

This book is written for you, whether as a person in the early stages of dementia or as a close friend or family member of someone facing dementia who is seeking answers and guidance. It is written in a manner to provide as close an experience as possible to speaking with me across my desk in the office—face to face, having an honest and sometimes difficult conversation. My patients are the center of every conversation, even if the treatment plan is directed toward a caregiver/care partner, spouse, or adult child who will help carry it out. This book is no different.

The brain and its diseases, such as dementia, tend to be mysterious and challenging for the scientific community and the public to understand. I wrote this book to pull back the curtain on how neurologic disorders like dementia continue to challenge our field and to help you better understand what we now know happens to the brain in dementia, how it affects you, and what we can do about it.

Doctors are responsible for the health of a large group of people and are informed by experience in direct care and research. This book serves as a means to that end, too, by enabling patients and families to become more informed about their health and learn how to plan ahead and handle any problems when they occur. This book cannot replace the conversations held between you and your own doctor when discussing dementia and is not a substitute for direct medical care. But it may serve as a reference for important points never discussed with your own doctor, a basis for asking more questions, and a resource on learning further about dementia.

Care needs in dementia can be addressed in many ways, and answers and advice should never come from the perspective of one physician. But the advice I give is based on years of experience in treating patients from diagnosis to treatment to hospice and death combined with the mentorship and expert training I received from many other physicians before me with decades of experience, supporting thousands of patients and families facing many of these same challenges. Built on this foundation, this book will help you better understand why this problem called dementia has developed and what lies ahead in order to develop a real-life road map to navigate life with dementia.

Throughout this text, I primarily refer to physicians and doctors directing care. Increasingly we rely on the dedicated efforts of nurse practitioners and physicians assistants, collectively known as "advance practice providers," to help deliver care. Many points in this book may be discussed with them, depending on their relationship to a neurological practice and general comfort with the subject matter.

Most science and clinical care is a team effort, and this book is no different. I would like to thank my family for their edits and support while I took time away from them to write this book. I thank my clinical staff and mentors at Columbia University Irving Medical Center (especially Drs. Karen Marder, John Brust, and Olajide Williams) for their constant support in everything that I do professionally; Ms. Carolyn Halpin-Healy of Arts & Minds for helping realize what else we can offer patients; and the patient editors of this book, including Mr. Craig Panner of Oxford University Press, Dr. Lisa Shulman (series editor), the superb editorial guidance of Ms. Debra Zoellner, and

Ms. Andrea Weiss of the American Academy of Neurology. But most important, I thank my patients, their families, and their caregivers for allowing me a window into their world and the opportunity to help them one visit at a time and for providing the foundation for development of this book intended for many more.

Introduction

Because you have opened this book, you or a close friend or family member have likely been impacted by the upsetting and frightening diagnosis of dementia. You may have been told about this diagnosis in a number of different ways. Either the term dementia was used, or other words associated with or more specific than dementia, such as Alzheimer's disease, vascular dementia, Lewy body disease, frontotemporal dementia, or Pick's disease, were used. You may even have been misinformed at first and told that you were simply facing the normal changes of aging, normal forgetfulness, or just mild depression. Sometimes these terms are relatable based on others we know who have been affected by them. But they can be shocking to hear and hard to understand when talking about yourself or a loved one. Even more difficult is that none of the most common forms of dementia currently have treatments that can cure or consistently slow the disease person to person.

This book begins by establishing a shared understanding of key terms used when describing dementia and explaining how dementia differs from the normal changes of aging. It then discusses the process of establishing a diagnosis, explains how the brain works in the process, and takes a deep dive into each of the most common types of dementia to help you understand them better. One of the hardest facts to begin to understand in dementia is that it is not diagnosed by a single test and is not usually found through routine screening. The journey leading to a diagnosis can be long and challenging and may even seem to lack a clear path forward. No two people experience dementia in the same way, and how a diagnosis is eventually established may vary based on the approach taken by different doctors or between centers. But giving a name to your experience is an important first step in discussing and validating your concerns and beginning to plan for the future.

The book then discusses treatments, including standard medical therapies for the symptoms of dementia, evolving treatments that target the biology of disease to potentially slow the course, and complementary strategies to support the patient and caregiver/care partner (sometimes also referred to as "carers"), as well as the option of participating in research. The changes that lie ahead and how to plan for the future are also explained. Throughout the book are patient stories to help you understand how problems may emerge in daily life. A glossary of terms is included at the back of the book to enhance learning, and glossary terms appear in boldface the first time they are mentioned. Helpful appendices at the end of the book include a list of vetted and reliable resources available for specific diseases and problems, tips on how to plan for a doctor visit, and information on participating in clinical trials. Whenever possible, a balance is struck between hope and realism, encouraging those with dementia and their loved ones to find joy despite contending with an often-terrible disease.

This book serves a dual purpose: to help in day-to-day challenges and in understanding what lies ahead. Reading straight through may be very upsetting and perhaps not appropriate; reading about late stages of disease at a time when you are contending with the earliest stages may not be immediately helpful but nonetheless will be important to understand eventually. Turn to sections addressing the problem before you, while trying to think just a few steps ahead. As you will discover, learning how to cope with, manage, and plan for this disease is a necessarily long process. Becoming more informed about dementia will help ground you during tough times. Try to stay focused on the type of care you want to give or receive.

No two persons with dementia are alike in presentation, course, symptom development, or duration. With dementia come unpredictable shifts in behavior, memory, and language developing slowly over time combined with sudden changes leading to unexpected challenges, such as sleepless nights, aggravation, denial, and depression. Trying to predict how someone may experience dementia is incredibly difficult and always an imperfect science. Most dementias will unfortunately worsen over time, but predictions about how quickly dementia may progress or what symptoms may arise first, if at all, may be imprecise or never come true. Dementia is a highly individualized experience.

Dementia will come to define nearly every aspect of life. Day-to-day routines will change, sometimes in unexpected ways and at unexpected times. Dementia affects the treatment of other illnesses, surgical decisions, prognoses, and follow-up plans. Friends and family may be called upon to become caregivers of an otherwise healthy person. Given the toll dementia can have on personal health, often in advanced age, dementia may also be the final chronic disease diagnosed in someone, which raises a whole host of important and unfortunately often overlooked issues related to palliative care.

A dementia diagnosis may challenge, change, and strain your family structure in many and unexpected ways, potentially over the course of many years. This is impossible to avoid, but this book can help you anticipate these changes and form a plan to address the challenges when they arise or even before they become real problems.

Dementia presents distinct challenges, including coping with its symptoms, finding resources and support, and figuring out how to anticipate behavioral and cognitive changes. However, it does not have to be overwhelming, even if difficult. This book is designed to provide guidance for the challenging steps of living with dementia as a patient, friend, or caregiver. The nature of most office visits highlights what individuals cannot do because of dementia. But whenever possible, this book focuses instead on what they *can* do, and most importantly what we all can do to better understand and treat dementia now and in the future.

CHAPTER 1

Dementia, Mild Cognitive Impairment, and Normal Changes of Aging

What's the Difference?

In this chapter, you will learn about:

- The answers to some of the most common foundational issues in dementia
- What the term dementia means
- What the term mild cognitive impairment, or MCI, means
- The differences between dementia, mild cognitive impairment, and normal changes of aging
- The fundamental concepts underlying a diagnosis of dementia or a related disorder

What is dementia?

This first chapter begins by reviewing answers to some of the most common big-picture questions asked of physicians, the first being "What is dementia?" **Dementia** is a collective, or "umbrella," term given to a group of diseases affecting the brain that cause someone to develop difficulty in thinking, speaking, remembering, or behaving in the way they did throughout their normal adult life. Dementia has recognizable **symptoms** (things felt, noticed, or experienced by the patient) and **signs** (problems identifiable to others, including family, friends, caregivers, or physicians). Although other words may describe changes in memory and thinking, the term dementia is used when these problems have started to change normal daily life routines. The somewhat newer term **major neurocognitive disorder** is used by some doctors but can be confusing and even more upsetting to hear than the term dementia, although it was developed, at least in part, to be a less stigmatizing term.

Age is an important factor in dementia, both in why some people may develop it and in how it is named. The terms early onset and late onset are used to describe the age when someone starts to have the first symptoms of dementia. A **late-onset dementia** typically refers to dementia that develops at age 60 years or later, whereas **early-onset dementia**, a far less common form, begins before age 60. Not to be confused with the onset of dementia, the terms early stage (or mild dementia), middle stage (moderate dementia), and late **stage** (severe dementia) may also be used to refer to how affected someone with dementia may be, irrespective of their age of onset. So someone can have early-onset or late-onset dementia and said to be in the early, middle, or late stage of dementia, regardless of their age of onset.

In dementia, problems with **memory**, **attention** and concentration, **processing speed**, **visuospatial** abilities, and language are referred to as **cognitive** symptoms. When these abilities of the brain are impacted, it is called **cognitive impairment**. Other changes, such as **depression**, anger, mood swings, or changes in personality, are referred to as **behavioral and psychological symptoms of dementia**, but you may also hear them referred to as **psychological, psychiatric**, or **neuropsychiatric symptoms** of dementia. Chapters 5 through 9 discuss the most common cognitive and behavioral findings in each of the most common forms of dementia.

The first signs and symptoms of dementia are often seen when people need help with chores, hobbies, or routine activities that are well known and have been part of their daily life for years. For people who are still working when symptoms develop, evidence of a decline in work performance may be seen or some form of assistance such as a new reminder system may be needed to accomplish an ordinary workload. Collectively, routine daily activities at home, work, or in the community are known as the **instrumental activities of daily living** (or **IADLs**), the many things we do independently on a daily basis, often without thinking about them. Of course, we all face new challenges each day, and sometimes we can't get them done. When one or several IADLs become difficult to accomplish, we may become aware of an emerging problem.

IADL tasks include but are not limited to:

- Managing personal finances, both monthly (i.e., bills), and annually (i.e., preparing taxes)
- Making a shopping list and fulfilling it accurately
- Planning and taking medications
- Attending appointments
- Preparing a meal
- Following the plot and characters of a television program or book
- Using common household appliances
- Traveling in familiar neighborhoods or navigating to new ones

This list of IADLs comes from research studies and may not fully capture an individual's specific abilities or needs. This list is also intended to pick up changes that are mainly caused by cognitive or memory problems and not those caused by physical problems. As an example, arthritis or a stroke may cause clumsiness or weakness but may have no impact on memory. Yet these physical problems may limit a person's ability to write or type or even open a pill bottle. Some of these tasks of daily living may be more relevant to some people than others, and some may not be obvious if the particular challenges are not part of daily life. For example, someone who takes no medications will not have problems with taking them, and someone who tends to stay close to home may not try new things. In these cases, changes won't be obvious. Another set of activities of daily living, the **basic** activities of daily living (BADLs), refer to other essential daily functions, such as personal hygiene (grooming and bathing), walking, eating, bathroom routines, and getting dressed. In contrast to IADLs, BADLs are usually impacted later in the course of dementia at a time when cognitive changes have become more obvious.

Some things that used to be considered as good indicators of cognitive changes have themselves changed. Much of life has shifted online, including banking and paying bills, which may be automated and less prone to errors than balancing a checkbook. Plus, it has become natural for people to use and even rely on smartphones as a part of daily life. One example is using a smartphone to help us with navigation while driving, making it hard to tell if someone has started to forget how to drive from one place to another. So it is not a change in any one individual IADL that is concerning, but an overall pattern makes us start to think about cognitive changes, especially changes that seem to be more than just those associated with aging itself.

What is mild cognitive impairment or predementia?

Before someone develops dementia with obvious changes in IADLs, most people pass through a transitional stage called **mild cognitive impairment**, or MCI. MCI is typically defined as a period of time when the person may notice some forgetfulness or other changes in thinking or behavior. In contrast to dementia, people with MCI still function at a fairly normal level; they can go to work, take care of most responsibilities in the home, and even provide care for other family members with complex needs. With the exception of a severe or sudden underlying change in the brain, such as might happen with a large stroke or severe brain trauma, most other forms of dementia begin with MCI.

Like dementia, MCI is a descriptive term that refers to a group of signs and symptoms and does not define the specific underlying biological cause. MCI also has a range of stages from the earliest (sometimes called early MCI or subjective cognitive impairment) to later stage MCI, when signs and symptoms are more apparent. MCI broadly falls into two main categories: **amnestic** and **nonamnestic.** Amnestic MCI refers to people who have forgetfulness (or amnesia, thus the term amnestic) as the main or most obvious cognitive symptom, although other problems in thinking may exist. Nonamnestic MCI means that, although someone has a cognitive problem greater than just what is expected for normal aging, memory is not really impaired or is not the primary issue.

For most age groups, having nonamnestic MCI without other neurologic problems carries the same or only slightly higher risk of developing dementia later on compared to the risk of age alone. But for many, amnestic MCI may be the same as the first symptoms of what will eventually become a more obvious dementia; it is thus an important distinction when considering care, including treatment, support, potential referral for diagnostic testing, and even research studies. Sometimes MCI, particularly nonamnestic MCI, improves, especially if a treatable or reversible cause of cognitive change is diagnosed (refer to Chapter 2 for further discussion on the diagnostic process). However, for many patients, MCI represents an important step in realizing a serious neurologic disease has started. Since a person with dementia will need care and assistance from others (**caregivers**), in MCI it is important to identify a **care partner** when planning ahead. Often care partners transition to becoming caregivers in the course of the disease.

When is it not just normal aging?

Aging itself is often blamed for changes in the way the brain works. There is great truth to this concept. Clearly, the brain works very differently at different stages of life, often purposefully. For instance, as a young child begins to acquire language, the capacity for memorizing passages in a book is impressive. Even before they can read, they can often recall lengthy book passages read to them, but this skill fades as reading evolves. Similarly, the skills of the aging mind differ with age. Older individuals have had more life experiences and more skill sets to draw upon when reviewing scenarios and considering outcomes. This is often referred to as wisdom, and, despite dementia, many people can continue to impart wisdom to others, often in brief but impressive and unexpected ways, even in later stages of disease.

The brain's ability to remember new information declines with aging. Many thousands of people have taken challenging thinking and memory tests in studies that show what is normal based on age, education history, and the principal language spoken. The results of these tests show what is within the range of normal cognitive aging. But when there is an inflection point—a noticeable change—in memory, concentration, attention, or language abilities, or when a substantially new personality trait develops, it may be the first sign of dementia.

To determine when that inflection point or transition started, consider the example of a question often asked on a birthday: "How does it feel to be 60?" Most would answer something along the lines of "about the same as yesterday when I was a year younger." In most forms of dementia, day-to-day changes are usually not noticeable, but year-to-year changes are. Figure 1.1 shows the continuum of changes between normal aging, MCI, and dementia.

Let's work through a few common scenarios to begin to understand the differences between dementia, MCI, and normal cognitive changes of aging.

Frank is a 78-year-old retired baker who lives with his wife of many years. Since his retirement 10 years ago, he and his wife have been constant companions at home and in their community. Their adult children are raising families of their own and only have a chance to get together every year for the winter

Normal cognitive aging	Mild cognitive impairment (MCI)	Dementia
• A range of changes in thinking and memory considered to be normal for age • Not an immediate precursor to MCI or dementia • Based on normative data across ages, languages, cultures	• A range of changes in thinking and memory NOT considered to be normal for age • Often a precursor for dementia • Without help, person remains independent in all regards	• A range of changes in thinking and memory NOT considered to be normal for age • Early: Person needs assistance in order to remain independent • Late: Person needs assistance in basic activities of daily living

FIGURE 1.1 **Progression of changes in normal aging, MCI, and dementia.** The cognitive and behavioral changes of normal cognitive aging, MCI, and dementia are distinct but occur on a continuum. The states are distinguished by both demonstrable changes and reliance on others for support.

holidays and some birthdays. During a visit, their daughter notices that her father cannot explain how to make his favorite bread recipe. Frank's wife steps in to help and explains that it is something that they started doing together a few years ago. Later in the conversation, Frank's daughter comes to realize he can't remember when she arrived and how long she has been there. He shares some of the same long-told family stories he has always shared over the holidays, but over the 2-day visit she hears the same story multiple times, sometimes twice in a single conversation. Frank's wife gets a little exasperated with hearing these same few stories he tells over and over now. She has explanations for the memory problems that have gradually worsened over time, but these changes are troubling to their daughter. A visit to their doctor to discuss memory loss is planned at their daughter's insistence.

Without a doubt, Frank has experienced obvious changes in his memory and other cognitive abilities. But it took their daughter visiting from out of town to make it clear to everyone around Frank that these changes are more than just the normal changes of aging. But sometimes these changes may not be obvious or may be hard to distinguish from the normal changes of aging.

Mabel is a 63-year-old anthropology professor who always had trouble learning the names of her students. She has otherwise been doing well professionally and even authored a new book last year. One day her husband notices that Mabel is having trouble recalling her new class schedule, even though it is a bit simpler than in prior semesters. Her physician recently changed the dose of her blood pressure medication only to find out she did not fill the new prescription. Her husband gets upset seeing these lapses in memory, but he has trouble determining whether they are just a few episodes that stand out to him or if they are part of a pattern of declining memory. When Mabel discussed her memory problems with colleagues or her husband, they all said it's just the problems they all deal with simply because they are getting older.

Although it may not be clear whether Mabel is experiencing MCI, the earliest signs of dementia, or just normal aging, what is clear is that she has experienced a change in her cognition and should be evaluated.

Carol, a 72-year-old woman, has been working as an architect in a large firm for many years. She is considered by others to be talented and leads projects that require complex design and creativity. However, over the past few years, her workload has increasingly shifted online, particularly communication with others. Following the recent retirement of her longtime design partner and the restructuring of her business, Carol increasingly needs to respond to e-mail messages and use new digital design software. She has difficulty learning the complex design programs that

> *younger professionals quickly master. She has also missed several*
> *important e-mails in the past few months. She does not think her*
> *work has been meaningfully affected but she decides to see a neur-*
> *ologist, who makes a tentative diagnosis of MCI.*

Whereas Frank has more obvious changes suggesting dementia and Mabel has subtle changes that are potentially normal for aging, Carol's declining memory is somewhere in the middle, and she probably has MCI.

Dementia, mild cognitive impairment, and Alzheimer's disease: how the terms fit together

What's the difference between dementia, MCI, and Alzheimer's disease? This is a question neurologists hear all the time, and it's a very valid question. In brief, the umbrella terms of MCI and dementia describe a person's signs and symptoms but not their diagnosis. A diagnosis more specifically describes the reasons why these symptoms developed.

Alzheimer's disease, which is discussed in detail in Chapter 5, is the most common form of dementia. This is why most people jump to this term when they hear the word "dementia" and assume that they have Alzheimer's disease. But dementia may have other causes, including dementia with Lewy bodies (Chapter 6), frontotemporal dementia (Chapter 7), and vascular dementia (Chapter 8), which refer to specific changes in the brain. Other less common causes of dementia are described in Chapter 9. The primary features and progression of each of the most common causes of dementia are presented in Table 1.1.

These changes that occur in the brain cells and in specific parts of the brain help us understand what type of dementia has developed. Each part of the brain has certain jobs or functions. When specific

TABLE 1.1 Primary Features of the Most Common Forms of Dementia

Name	Primary features	Progression
Alzheimer's disease (Chapter 5)	Memory loss for recent events, word-finding difficulty, visuospatial problems, low interest in activities, anger and irritability, denial of a problem, sundowning	Slowly progressive over years
Dementia with Lewy bodies (Chapter 6)	Memory loss and visuospatial disorientation; physical changes, including tremor, slowness, stiffness, and imbalance (parkinsonism); visual hallucinations and misperceptions; dream enactment	Slowly progressive over years; severity may vary day to day
Frontotemporal dementia (Chapter 7)	Changes in personality, language, or memory, which may be accompanied by parkinsonism or, less often, motor neuron disease (amyotrophic lateral sclerosis)	Slowly progressive over years
Vascular dementia (Chapter 8)	Any of the above features; may be accompanied by weakness or language problems after an obvious stroke	Stepwise decline over years; may have sudden or obvious changes following a large stroke
Other less common causes of dementia (Chapter 9)	Varies depending on diagnosis, and includes signs and symptoms specific to Huntington's disease, Creutzfeldt–Jakob disease, normal pressure hydrocephalus, and dementia associated with brain tumors, epilepsy, and multiple sclerosis	Varies, depending on the diagnosis

areas are affected, the associated pattern of cognitive and behavioral problems helps to determine the diagnosis.

When does MCI or dementia begin?

As demonstrated in the cases described earlier, identifying when MCI or dementia begins can be hard to determine, especially since normal changes of thinking and memory occur with aging. Some health problems, such as heart attack or stroke, have a clear and sudden onset so the date and even exact time of onset of symptoms can be determined. Sometimes cognitive changes in dementia are obvious, such as the first time someone gets lost in their own neighborhood. But as a rule, the early cognitive changes preceding dementia are subtle and insidious and are often explained away as just aging.

For example, it may be unreasonable to expect someone to easily begin to use a computer late in life. But that is just what is increasingly asked of us. Banks, insurance companies, and doctors' offices expect older adults to adapt to managing their lives online even if they don't have the skills or experience. So, it can be difficult to determine whether someone's inability to use a computer is of concern. A question to consider is whether the inability reflects new cognitive problems and the onset of dementia or is simply less cognitive flexibility and a general reluctance to change. On the other hand, when someone has used a computer for many years and then becomes unable to do so, that is a time for concern. Similarly, when someone has trouble remembering a frequently used login ID or a commonly used password or bank PIN, that should begin to raise concern. And if someone suddenly can't understand how to set up a new password or even take the first steps to resolve this problem, it is also a troubling sign of a change in **cognition,** a broad term used to describe thinking, memory, perception, or language function of the brain.

The first symptoms and signs of dementia may become apparent in some people with emerging dementia far earlier in the course of the illness than others. For example, people with difficult jobs requiring good memory and multitasking abilities may show obvious signs early when they can no longer multitask or when they forget where their files are located. Dementia can begin to impact work because of forgetfulness, inattention, poor concentration, difficulty in planning, or personality changes. In contrast, during retirement people have fewer day-to-day responsibilities and high-stakes decisions are uncommon. When less is asked of us on a day-to-day basis, a more substantial change in cognition may be necessary for dementia to become obvious to others. Just as the symptoms of dementia begin gradually and slowly over a long time, so do the changes in the brain cells leading to dementia; these changes may take place over years before the first symptoms are noticed.

> ### *Take-home point*
>
> *Dementia represents a meaningful change in how the brain works such that daily functions are affected and cannot be accomplished independently.*

Snapshots in time versus the long view

Friends or family members in frequent daily contact may not notice subtle slow changes over time. In contrast, someone who visits infrequently may notice substantial changes, as they have the ability to compare two visits separated by a substantial time gap. The closer we are to someone, the harder it may be to see or recognize changes. The daily cognitive changes seen by a spouse or close friend may not be as obvious as the changes seen by an adult child who lives far away and can only compare snapshot-like visits over time, such as when visiting someone for a holiday from one year to the next.

Seeing an obvious change versus looking for it

Often, concern for dementia comes after a life-changing event such as the death of a spouse, a medical illness or surgery requiring hospitalization, a major financial transaction, or moving to a new home. In the moment, it can be easy to blame these major life events for cognitive change, and perhaps reasonably so. They are all highly stressful, and stress changes the way people act and remember, no matter what their age. But during these stressful events, those with cognitive problems are often watched more closely or get more attention from others. The death of a spouse may suddenly reveal how much the pair relied on one another; sometimes in aging couples, one serves a physical role (lifting, carrying, taking out the trash), while the other takes on all things requiring memory and **executive skills** (medications, bills, and appointments). A hospitalization may bring family members to the bedside, causing them to recognize frailty and memory loss. Hospitalization can also reveal how difficult being away from home can be or how susceptible someone is to a minor change in routine or medication side effects. Moving to a new home may help with mobility problems but may reveal an unexpected problem with learning new things, such as how to get around a new home or neighborhood.

After a major life event for someone with cognitive problems, a close and observant family member may begin to more closely monitor cognitive and behavioral changes. Ultimately, these observations may be brought to the attention of a primary care physician or may generate a referral to a neurologist. Adding further to the challenge of establishing the onset of dementia, about half of people with dementia are unaware of their cognitive problems to some degree or even altogether. Recognizing these problems often requires the observation of others.

Wendy is 58 years old and works as an office cleaner in a high-rise office building. She is brought to the attention of a physician after she was fired. She accidentally entered a busy office meeting to clean the room and then repeatedly reentered despite multiple requests to leave. She has been an exemplary employee by accounts of her supervisors. However, one of her friends at work tells Wendy's husband that Wendy has not actually been doing her job well and has needed more instruction and supervision over the past 2 years, especially the past 6 months. She worked the night shift for many years and seldom saw her family except on the weekends or vacation. A review of her cognitive function with extended family reveals that major cognitive changes had been noticed at recent family gatherings when she forgot important ingredients of her favorite recipes. All of these changes were attributed to inadequate sleep, but this had not improved despite the change to a more normal sleep schedule.

Take-home point

The timing of the onset of dementia can be very difficult to determine, and it may only be recognized in retrospect using multiple perspectives from people with both daily and infrequent interactions with the person with dementia. It is important to note these problems when they occur and bring them to your doctor's attention.

Understanding the patient's perspective

Different approaches to understanding dementia are presented throughout this book through the lenses of scientists, physicians, caregivers, and those experiencing dementia during its earliest changes. But is also important to understand the person at the center of it all and how they experience dementia throughout its course. Doing so can give us insight into how to best provide care.

Imagine walking into a room, having a conversation, reading a book, following a television program, going to a doctor's appointment, or trying to take your daily medications while experiencing memory loss. Throughout our lifetimes, we are generally able to remember the sequence of events that led to the present moment, with the most recent steps in this sequence being most vivid in detail. Now try to imagine what it would be like if at this very moment, you were unable to recall what happened over an hour ago, 30 minutes ago, 5 minutes ago, or 30 seconds ago. Certainly, we have all had lapses in memory and been unable to recall some of the unimportant details of events that happened days or weeks ago. The normal function of memory is imperfect, designed to retain the most important and emotionally relevant information to guide one's path day to day. Some days we may have trouble remembering some things, possibly because of stress, poor sleep, or being preoccupied. But imagine the experience of trying to recall what happened just minutes ago, but you can't. And now imagine having that feeling often, every day, day after day, week after week, month after month. And what's more, now imagine that this problem gets worse and progresses over time.

Understanding how the brain attempts to compensate for memory lapses helps us understand common responses to cognitive problems such as forgetfulness. Take, for example, the common scenario of misplacing keys or losing a wallet. For most of us, misplacing the keys is simply a consequence of being preoccupied when the keys are thrown onto the first flat surface encountered in our home. After retracing our steps or searching a few of the most likely places they could be, the keys are found and the memory of how the keys were misplaced is recalled. Most important, we understand the most likely explanation: a busy and tiresome end to the day.

In contrast, when a wallet is permanently lost, reasonable explanations may be few and may include theft, especially in a busy urban environment. For most people with normal memory, attributing loss to theft is a very reasonable explanation and one that would be supported by other family members and friends. For someone with dementia who is unaware that they have memory loss, the most reasonable explanation for a lost wallet may still be that it was stolen. However, a person with dementia is less likely to consider other scenarios, such as the wallet being left on a restaurant table or grocery store checkout counter, and instead presumes theft. This example highlights how a common experience may give rise to unrealistic interpretations, anxiety, and agitation.

From this perspective, the emotional impact of frequently feeling confused and forgetful without any explanation may be recognized. For many with dementia, this can be a desperate feeling, but it can be helped when care partners anticipate the situations that contribute to these misperceptions, and recognize when emotions, irritability, and anger begin to escalate. Many people with dementia fail to recognize the problems and have little insight but are not prone to agitation, anger, or paranoia. Learning to address and anticipate a stressful situation is essential. Anticipating or averting a stressful situation or emotional response is always the preferred route, as options for treatment are somewhat limited or incompletely effective.

By appreciating the difficulties experienced by people with dementia, ways to anticipate, address, and prevent some of their distressing behavioral responses can be learned. All too often, loving caregivers become distressed or angry with the individual experiencing dementia, challenging them to understand a situation or perform a cognitive task that can no longer be accomplished. This reaction is, to some degree, natural. If someone does not remember something, how another tries to get them to remember by any means, gentle or aggressive, may even be part of a long-standing manner by which two individuals interact. These dynamics may be ingrained among husband and wife, parent and child, or close friends for many years.

Family and friends face the difficult task of adjusting to a new set of rules and expectations. The cognitive, behavioral, and emotional problems that the spouse, parent, or friend is experiencing are simply beyond their control. Confronting the person with dementia about their behavior seldom has any benefit, often leads to anger between the person with dementia and caregiver, and escalates anxiety and agitation. One must recognize that they are dealing with a disease and not an individual doing something on purpose.

> ### Take-home point
>
> *Don't get angry at the person with dementia. Their behavior is beyond their control. Focus your energy on controlling the symptoms of the disease, not arguing with the person with dementia.*

Without a doubt, learning about a new diagnosis of dementia is stressful and can be overwhelming. It is normal to be upset when thinking about dementia in someone we know. You are not alone. The next chapters in this book explain how dementia is diagnosed, how the brain is changed by the different causes of dementia, and, most important, what to do about it.

CHAPTER 2

Diagnosing Dementia

In this chapter, you will learn about:

- The steps physicians take to make a diagnosis of dementia, including taking a history and conducting a neurologic examination
- Standard diagnostic tests that are used to identify potentially treatable or reversible causes of dementia
- Biomarker-based tests, including imaging and cerebrospinal fluid (CSF) analyses, that can clarify the underlying cause of dementia
- The role of specialists in the process of establishing a diagnosis, including dementia-focused neurologists, neuropsychologists, and genetic counselors

As described in Chapter 1, the central questions that patients, families, and physicians face are similar: Does the person have dementia, mild cognitive impairment (MCI), or normal changes of aging? Or is there another medical reason for the cognitive problems? And, if the diagnosis is dementia or MCI, what is the underlying cause? These questions guide the path toward a diagnosis. This chapter reviews the steps a physician will take in connecting signs and symptoms of disease with the underlying biology.

The diagnostic process can take time and is imperfect. How some of the most common causes of dementia are diagnosed is changing and reflects ongoing scientific advances in the field. Some new tools doctors have to diagnose dementia have become more and more accurate in recent years. It is hoped that the ability to now make a very specific diagnosis will help in the future when new disease-specific treatments become available.

Establishing the exact diagnosis in Alzheimer's disease, dementia with Lewy bodies, frontotemporal dementia, vascular dementia, and other forms of dementia can be challenging. For the most part, an exact dementia diagnosis cannot be made by any single part of the history (when the doctor asks the patient and family a number of questions) or examination, a blood test, or a brain scan. Currently, neurologists rely upon the history and examination to align with the additional tests, which often support the story but sometimes lead in unexpected directions, revealing new and possibly treatable problems. Unlike other problems that require medical care, such as high blood pressure (which is easy to measure) and common infections that are easy to detect, a dementia diagnosis is uncertain and unique. Although some brain scans can pick up important brain changes years before problems might start, those tests do not tell us the whole story of how someone is affected now. Some people can have very abnormal laboratory test results or brain scans but lead completely normal lives.

Simple, definitive, and noninvasive tests to diagnose dementia (such as a blood test) are just now starting to become available in the field of dementia, particularly those that can confirm a diagnosis of Alzheimer's disease. In past few decades, research has focused on making a diagnosis based on evidence of brain changes down to the microscopic level by the least invasive means possible, and these tests are finally becoming available. The hope is that by picking up on brain changes, which may begin years or even a decade or more before the first symptoms start, new treatments can begin to be found for dementia to prevent cognitive changes from happening in the first place. For now, the focus remains on clinical evaluations of current symptoms and how to manage them, but the shift toward identifying a cause of dementia that can be diagnosed and tracked through imaging and bloodwork has begun.

Cognitive problems exist on a spectrum, with the normal changes of aging on one end, dementia on the other, and MCI in the middle ground. The physician will evaluate each concern discussed, noting how severe the problems are, how often they are noticed, how long they have been present, and how they impact life. This is part of the history, or initial examination, that will be performed when the patient suspects something is wrong. The specific type or form of dementia (the underlying cause) is then diagnosed based on the pattern of signs and symptoms that emerge over the course of dementia, the mix of cognitive and behavioral problems, the timing and pace of progression, changes that may have occurred in mobility and movement, and a handful of additional diagnostic tests.

Step 1: It starts with a doctor's visit

Diagnosing what has caused dementia can be challenging throughout the course of disease, especially in the latest stages when all forms look similar. Doctors may follow the following common sequence of events to make a diagnosis, but everyone's path will differ.

History

No matter the medical situation when going to a doctor (or seeing one online by telehealth) for a dementia evaluation or anything else, physicians first develop an approach to making a diagnosis by taking a history. The vast majority of what the doctor needs to know can be learned simply by listening to the person (and caregiver/care partner or family member) and detailing a relevant history from when the first symptom was noticed to the present time. Physicians begin thinking about a list of likely diagnoses based on the history. In the case of possible dementia, the doctor will ask questions about whether there have been any changes in memory, concentration, language, visual skills, and **mood**; when each problem began; and what has happened over the course of time since the first hints of changes began.

Questions asked in clarifying the history aim to determine the duration of symptoms, the pattern of changes (slow or fast, static or progressive, or episodic changes), the earliest and most pervasive **cognitive** changes, evidence of changes in **behavior**, and the presence or absence of changes in physical function, including **gait, tremor**, slowness, weakness, imbalance, and/or falls. A detailed behavioral history will explore if the person has had any change in mood or personality, changes in energy levels or appetite, loss of interest in doing certain things, or changes in sleep habits. Identifying the pattern of changes, including how these changes may have become apparent relative to one another over time or how they may relate to mood, can be highly informative in determining a diagnosis. Additional questions will also be asked to determine if dementia is a common disease in late life in other close family members. The doctor will also ask questions about health habits (such as smoking and drinking alcohol), any drug abuse, and years of education and professional histories.

The doctor may have difficulty reconciling some parts of the history. For example, it may be unclear whether a recent period of depression is another episode in a lifelong history of depression or an early symptom of dementia. This is important to clarify, as changes in personality and mood may be an early sign of dementia.

Ideally, the history is provided by the affected person and someone who knows them well, typically a close family member or friend. Talking about these problems, especially changes in memory or personality, can be very upsetting and stressful, especially if the concerns don't make sense to the person experiencing the described changes. Moreover, the person with dementia may forget or be unaware of their own problems. It is important to be honest and open with the doctor as they take a history. This can become a problem if someone does not remember the reasons for a doctor's evaluation and the only things discussed are symptoms that seem wrong or unfamiliar to the person with cognitive impairment. How patients interact with others during the history-taking process can also be very informative, including disagreements, unexpected reactions to things said, or even how often the patient turns to a loved one to help provide information they can't remember or say.

Charlie is a 71-year-old man who is accompanied by his 46-year-old son David on a visit to his doctor. David decided to make a special appointment with his father's doctor based on his concerns about memory lapses over the past 6 months. At first, the memory lapses happened once in a while, but they have become increasingly noticeable on a daily basis. David tells the doctor that a few months ago Charlie repeated the same questions in conversation, but more recently he has forgotten an entire day's events. Sometimes when David points this out, Charlie gets upset; even when discussing the topic in the office, Charlie quickly becomes dismissive of David's concerns, chalking it up to normal changes of aging. Charlie otherwise thinks his memory is just fine, although he couldn't explain why he had not followed his doctor's recent instruction to take a new blood pressure medication and had missed recent appointments with his cardiologist and ophthalmologist. During an examination of memory, Charlie turns to David for help with the answers to the doctor's questions. Based on the history, examination findings, and the way Charlie responds to David's concerns, the doctor begins the diagnostic process for dementia.

Unfortunately, cognitive impairment can be overlooked in the primary care setting, perhaps because doctors have an obligation to address many other important health issues during the visit, limited time is available to screen for cognitive impairment, and the fact that about half of forgetful persons are unaware of their symptoms. That is, about half of all forgetful persons forget that they forget. Someone who is unaware of memory problems and goes unaccompanied to doctor visits is much more likely to have a delay in dementia diagnosis, even if symptoms are becoming obvious at home. To avoid this potential problem, every effort should be made to have someone accompany a person who has or is at risk for cognitive problems to their doctor visits to explain any concerns.

If it is uncomfortable to share concerning parts of the history in front of friends or family, this information can be provided to the physician in the form of a letter in advance of the visit or given to the doctor as part of the intake paperwork. This approach can help the doctor review potentially sensitive matters in a supportive way. It is important to be concise in such letters, prioritize needs, and ask for specific solutions to the problems demanding the most attention. Problems should be categorized as specifically as possible, including the type of problem, time of day it occurs, whether it is frequent or infrequent, and whether it is bothersome or not. If a summary letter cannot be provided, family and caregivers can work with a physician or their staff to briefly discuss major concerns in advance of the joint patient–family visit. In dementia, the neurologic history and examination have proven very adaptable to telehealth and virtual visits.

Examination

After the history is obtained, a physical examination provides information complementary to the history and serves to refine the approach to a diagnosis. The actual examination is composed of two major components, the **general medical examination** and the **neurologic examination**, and serves several purposes: (1) to confirm reported symptoms and your doctor's initial impressions based on the history, (2) to reveal new findings not readily apparent from the history, and (3) to investigate problems that may be unresolved following the history.

The general medical examination is probably familiar to most people as it is part of routine medical visits; it includes assessments of the eyes, ears, neck, heart, lungs, abdomen, arms, and legs. Some aspects of the general medical examination will serve to exclude unrecognized and possible contributing factors, such as stroke.

The neurologic examination focuses on the elements of the **nervous system** and takes a closer look at sensation, muscle strength and movement, reflexes, balance, and gait (how someone walks). The neurologic examination is quite observational and really begins when the patient enters the doctor's office, which can reveal changes in how someone walks, follows simple instructions, and interacts with others. With the expansion of virtual care during the COVID-19 pandemic, the same points apply to online evaluations, both in history and examination. Specific to a dementia evaluation, the neurologic examination will focus on testing for cognitive and behavioral changes. The main goal of a dementia examination is to identify cognitive, behavioral, and physical problems and determine how the findings connect with the history. The cognitive examination includes assessments of orientation, or how aware the patient is of the current time and place. Memory is assessed by asking the patient to remember a few words or a sentence for a few minutes or information from long ago and by how well current events are known. Language testing involves asking the patient to name common things, repeat phrases, follow a series of commands, and read and write. Tests of attention and concentration or **executive skills** determine how well the patient can think about several things at once or shift between one idea and another. Visuospatial abilities are assessed by asking the patient to draw or copy a picture. Other tests assess processing speed and reaction time. Overall, a screening cognitive assessment takes just a few minutes and can be instructive. But what is clear is that no one test tells the whole story, and everybody performs differently on these tests, whether or not a cognitive problem is suspected. When interpreting these tests, doctors take into consideration how someone might have performed on these tests even before problems began. These tests are imperfect but nonetheless can be helpful in picking up on cognitive problems more formally than just the history.

Putting together the information learned from the history and examination, the doctor mentally puts together a list of the most likely diagnoses underlying the symptoms and tries to determine what (if any) can't-miss, life-threatening diagnoses should be considered too. If dementia is suspected, the doctor will be concerned principally about Alzheimer's disease or, less commonly, dementia with Lewy bodies, frontotemporal dementia, or vascular dementia. The doctor will also want to make sure that the history and examination don't suggest something needing urgent attention, such as a developing tumor or recent stroke.

Step 2: Common tests ordered after initial evaluation

At the conclusion of the history and examination, the doctor will usually order several tests that focus on refining the diagnosis or excluding possible reversible causes that are, unfortunately, relatively infrequent. Most doctors will screen for reversible causes of dementia through bloodwork and imaging.

Possible reversible causes of cognitive problems include problems with the **thyroid gland**, **metabolic disorders** affecting the kidney or liver, **vitamin deficiencies** (especially vitamin B_{12}), or infections (including **HIV** and, rarely, **syphilis**). These can all be assessed through blood work, or **phlebotomy**. Although uncommon, prior exposure to syphilis can cause memory problems. If blood is being checked for syphilis, the doctor is not judging in any way; it is just a fact of life that the infection is still around and many people have been exposed, often without knowledge for many years. Rarely, it can cause dementia and is worth identifying since it might be treatable. Some other rare causes of rapid presentations of dementia may lead the doctor to conduct other blood tests as needed.

Rarely, something will be discovered in the course of the diagnostic process that will lead the diagnostic approach in another direction; even more rarely, this new finding may change the underlying diagnosis. Sometimes the workup may reveal a previously unrecognized medical problem, such as poor thyroid or kidney function, that results in dementia symptoms earlier than would have occurred otherwise. When the metabolic problems are corrected, the dementia symptoms may go away, at least for some months. Often, dementia symptoms may come back, even when the metabolic problem is resolved.

Along with these blood laboratory tests, a brain scan such as a **computed tomography** (**CT**) **scan** (or "cat" scan) or, alternatively, **magnetic resonance imaging** (**MRI**) will be suggested. Generally, an MRI is preferred as it tells more about the brain, and, although infrequent, imaging can show a previously unrecognized problem such as a stroke or brain tumor that was not otherwise apparent on history or examination. But sometimes an MRI cannot be done because the person has claustrophobia or a metal or implanted medical device (such as some heart pacemakers) that don't allow for an MRI. In these cases, a CT can provide the most important information. Basic laboratory and imaging evaluations can be accomplished at most testing centers with enough consistency and reliability for the physician.

In recent years, it has also become recognized that structural brain imaging (like that described earlier) can identify specific patterns of change in the shape or contour of the brain that can help refine the diagnostic approach. Subtle patterns in the shape, size, and contour of the brain may suggest a pattern typical of certain types of dementia. **Atrophy**, or shrinkage, of the brain is commonly seen with aging, but when it is more pronounced than expected or when it affects certain brain regions more than others, the regions of brain affected by atrophy can help inform the diagnosis. The typical changes of atrophy in Alzheimer's disease are shown in Figure 2.1.

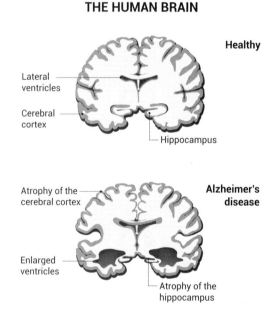

THE HUMAN BRAIN

FIGURE 2.1 **Brain atrophy in Alzheimer's disease.** Brain atrophy, or brain shrinkage, occurs over time with aging and in regionally specific patterns in neurodegenerative causes of dementia, including Alzheimer's disease. Shown here in a side to side view are the main changes of atrophy throughout the brain, especially in the hippocampus (which is essential for establishing new memory). The brain's ventricles expand into the new space left behind as the brain itself shrinks. Changes like these are seen on a CT or MRI of the brain.

Except in cases of stroke or tumor, MRIs and CTs usually cannot tell us what changes have happened in recent days or weeks; rather, they show us the changes that have accumulated over many months to years. Because the brain changes typically take place over the course of years, an MRI or CT done early in the course of illness is usually the only one that will be needed and it is not necessary to repeat the imaging except in special circumstances. With aging, separate and new neurologic problems can occur, such as a stroke, and another MRI or CT may be performed then.

Additional tests may be suggested to help with the workup at this stage. As an example, if the person is not sleeping well, a sleep study (**polysomnogram**) may be ordered, especially if a diagnosis of **sleep apnea** is possible. Sleep apnea is quite common; it is seen in people who snore loudly, have headaches, and readily fall asleep during the day and is associated with executive cognitive problems.

Howard is an 82-year-old retired mathematician whose wife has noticed that he can't keep track of the right day to take out the trash and recycling. She has written this down for them both on a calendar posted in the kitchen, and more recently she has reminded him of the date too. At his regularly scheduled annual physical examination with his primary care physician, his wife brings this problem to the doctor's attention and has summarized her concerns over time in a letter shared at the visit. Howard's doctor asks a series of questions about how long this has been going on and whether Howard has had any changes in memory, sleep, mood, and driving skill. A thorough physical examination is performed and reveals only that Howard cannot provide the date or details of recent news events or retain three words told to him several minutes before. A workup for dementia is started by their primary care physician, beginning with basic laboratory tests and a brain MRI.

> *Take-home point*
>
> To get the highest yield out of a visit with a primary care phys-
> ician, be prepared. Come to the visit with specific questions and
> objectives, knowing that the physician may explore other issues
> in dementia that need to be discussed.

Step 3: Referral to a neurologist or other specialist in dementia

At some point during or even before this step of the workup, the primary care physician may recommend that the patient see a **neurologist** to help with the diagnostic workup or treatment. Some
families begin by seeing a neurologist, which can be helpful, but
may then miss out on the important coordinating role served by a
primary care physician. Unfortunately, wait times to see a neurologist are often long. Telehealth may help address access to neurologic
and dementia specialty care. For uncomplicated cases of dementia,
many primary care physicians will be responsible for diagnosis and
management for much of the course and may only refer patients to
a neurologist when atypical or unusual features emerge or when a
second opinion is needed. Practices are adapting to newly available
treatments in Alzheimer's disease that need the guidance of experienced neurologists (Chapter 10). Other common reasons for referral
to a neurologist for dementia include a questionable or unsettled diagnosis; atypical features, including young age, rapid decline, seizures,
and features of Parkinson's disease (Chapter 6); severe agitation and
disruptive behaviors; sleep disturbances; and the need for medication
adjustments to manage these problems.

   A neurologist is a physician with knowledge of general medical problems and specialty training in neurologic diseases, including dementia and other disorders of cognitive impairment. Some

neurologists may have special experience, training, or qualifications in dementia. These dementia-focused neurologists may be identified as specializing in geriatric neurology or behavioral neurology and neuropsychiatry. Some **psychiatrists**, including geriatric psychiatrists, may have related expertise and experience in dementia. These specialists practice in a range of locations, from private practices to academic centers. An evaluation for dementia by a neurologist is usually done in an outpatient office and, like the examination performed by the primary care physician, includes reviewing the history and conducting an examination.

A neurologist will explore certain aspects of the history from their neurologically focused perspective and may be more attuned to determining a precise underlying diagnosis through additional testing, including more in-depth cognitive and behavioral assessments called **neuropsychological testing**. Additionally, a neurologist (or even the primary care physician) may recommend additional **biomarker** studies, which aim to make as precise a diagnosis as possible of what is happening to the brain cells. The neurologist is also typically the physician who directs the more complicated management decisions in certain stages of dementia, often in collaboration with the primary care physician. Beyond the initial workup and management, neurologists, especially those with expertise in dementia, may be best able to connect people with dementia to local patient and caregiver support resources and refer them to research studies if they are interested. Discussed later in this book in further detail are management (Chapters 10, 11, and 12), advance care planning (Chapter 15), and research (Appendix D).

Neuropsychological testing

In addition to cognitive evaluations, patients may be referred for formal neuropsychological testing. Similar to an examination in the doctor's office, neuropsychological testing explores the patient's memory, executive function, language, and visuospatial abilities and includes behavioral assessments. But these evaluations go into greater depth and they are performed by a **neuropsychologist**. A neuropsychologist is someone who holds a doctorate (Ph.D.) in neuropsychology and has expertise in test selection, delivery, and interpretation. Neuropsychologists perform and interpret these tests and may provide feedback, counseling, and even diagnosis, but they do not prescribe medications. More broadly, psychologists are non-physician clinicians who often work closely with psychiatrists to treat persons with mood problems through counseling. Psychologists are not often a part of dementia care given that psychological care requires both insight and intact memory. However, psychologists can be essential in treating distressed caregivers or persons with memory problems specifically due to depression or anxiety. Many neuropsychologists serve in the roles of psychologists, offering therapy and counseling in addition to diagnostic assessments.

Neuropsychological evaluations usually take several hours, although they may be shorter (or occasionally take place over several visits) at the discretion of the neuropsychologist. Neuropsychological testing is most informative when done early in the course of illness so that specific domains of cognitive abilities can be tested and compared against one another. Automated computerized neuropsychological testing may be suggested in some centers, and telehealth/virtual options are becoming increasingly available. Although these tests tend to be shorter and more convenient than formal neuropsychological testing, such automation can lack the nuance required of some evaluations as well as the skilled interpretation offered by neuropsychologists. Not everyone has access to a neuropsychologist, but often these assessments are preferred over automated testing by both patient and doctor.

Neuropsychological testing provides important information that a simple office-based assessment cannot. It helps understand how patients perform relative to their peers (typically matched by age and level of education) and through metrics that can estimate what the expected performance would have been before any memory problems began. Such testing may not be needed in moderate to severe cognitive impairment, as it may not be particularly helpful by that stage. Unlike the diagnostic tests discussed earlier, neuropsychological test performance and interpretation can vary substantially between providers based upon experience and expertise. If available, it is important to work with someone with experience in the field of aging and dementia.

Once neuropsychological tests are completed, typically within a few days or weeks, findings are reviewed in a return visit with the neuropsychologist or neurologist. Taken together, the history and examination, laboratory work, imaging, and neuropsychological testing can help answer key questions:

- Where on the spectrum of normal aging to MCI to dementia are the patient's current problems (Chapter 1)?
- What seems to be the most likely reason for the symptoms?
- Is the condition treatable and/or reversible?

The next section moves beyond describing the clinical syndrome/problem and into why it is happening.

Step 4: Using biomarkers to make the diagnosis

Overall, the pattern of cognitive problems identified through office-based assessments and neuropsychological testing can help in understanding whether the pattern matches the normal changes of aging or if the changes are what would be expected in MCI or dementia. Once a diagnosis of MCI or dementia is suggested by the workup and most other medical problems have been ruled out, the physicians will try to further refine the diagnosis of dementia into one of the underlying causes. However, precise diagnosis continues to be a great challenge in the field. Many of the common causes of dementia, such as Alzheimer's disease (Chapter 5), dementia with Lewy bodies (Chapter 6), and frontotemporal dementia (Chapter 7), have overlapping clinical features.

The different types of dementia can look very similar in daily life yet are very different when considered on a **microscopic** level. Currently, the only way to make an exact diagnosis of the type of dementia is by looking at the brain tissue of the affected person under the microscope, which, of course, isn't possible during any doctor visits. Each type of dementia has its own hallmarks seen under the microscope involving the abnormal aggregation, or clumping, of special brain proteins. Yet some microscopic findings overlap between forms of dementia, and it is increasingly recognized that the microscopic picture can be different from person to person even when the same disease is diagnosed.

One way to obtain a microscopic picture of the brain is by a brain **biopsy**, a surgical sampling of a small amount of brain tissue. Most people with dementia will not need a biopsy, except in highly unusual presentations. Sometimes biopsies are done to clarify why someone has very rapid progression, which, in rare cases, may indicate a cause that is treatable to slow, stop, or even reverse the changes seen.

A brain **autopsy**, including a microscopic analysis of the whole brain, is done after death and remains the only way of definitively knowing what kind of changes occurred in the brain and what caused the dementia. For the most part, postmortem studies are performed at large research centers. While, of course, an autopsy cannot help an individual living person, brain autopsies have helped researchers make important strides in better understanding the disease in general. An autopsy can also provide a definitive answer and some closure for families. Increasingly, other measures called biomarkers, which use other tests to indirectly diagnose dementia based on what is happening in the cells of the brain, are being relied on for diagnosis.

Advanced diagnostic techniques: using biomarkers to diagnose dementia

Biomarkers are measurements that can help doctors determine the cause of dementia. Currently, advanced brain imaging techniques and CSF analyses can be used to identify dementia biomarkers. Of course, great interest exists in making diagnosis less invasive, such as through a blood test; tests like these are just starting to become available, particularly to diagnose Alzheimer's disease. In the meantime, other biomarkers are helpful in distinguishing the underlying cause of dementia when someone has signs and symptoms. Biomarkers are commonly used in research studies to identify preclinical signs of dementia (before any symptoms begin) but are generally not recommended for use in healthy individuals. With the availability of new treatments for Alzheimer's disease, biomarkers are expected to take on an increasingly important role in establishing or confirming the cause of dementia. Since it is likely that most treatments targeting the biological changes of progressive dementias are more effective when given as early as possible, a biomarker-based diagnoses of dementia will become increasingly important in the diagnostic process.

Nuclear medicine neuroimaging

Nuclear medicine studies are used to diagnose dementia by showing whether the brain and its cells (neurons) show changes suggestive of certain types of dementia. The most commonly used nuclear medicine studies are **positron emission tomography** (**PET**) and **single-photon emission computed tomography** (**SPECT**). Three kinds of PET exist: one tagged with a glucose or sugar molecule, fluorodeoxyglucose (**FDG-PET**), and others with a protein such as amyloid (**amyloid PET**) or tau (**tau PET**). Brain SPECT testing in dementia measures brain perfusion or blood flow. Low sugar metabolism or low perfusion can suggest brain problems when they occur in certain patterns involving the parts of the brain affected by

Alzheimer's disease, frontotemporal dementia, or, possibly, dementia with Lewy bodies. Although the tests are not perfect, they can be very helpful if they are clearly normal or clearly fit a pattern of dementia such as Alzheimer's disease. A special type of SPECT scan is called a **dopamine transporter (DaT) scan**; it focuses on the deep structures of the brain involved in parkinsonism. DaT scans may be useful in diagnosing dementia with Lewy bodies.

Newer to the field of dementia are the protein-specific amyloid PET and tau PET scans. In contrast to showing brain function, these scans identify if and where the abnormal proteins are being deposited in the brain—the same proteins seen under the microscope following a biopsy or autopsy. Thus, these tests can show if someone has changes consistent with Alzheimer's disease or one of a few other related disorders. It is hoped that in the near future, PET imaging or other noninvasive tests (such as bloodwork) will be able to make a biological basis of dementia diagnosis for all. Moreover, these and other techniques hold promise to establish a diagnosis when brain changes have occurred but before symptoms begin. With the availability of **disease-modifying therapy** for Alzheimer's disease (medicines that can impact the primary microscopic changes in dementia, covered further in Chapter 10), these tests help guide treatment early in the course of disease. Further details on nuclear medicine imaging are provided in Appendix A.

Cerebrospinal fluid analyses

It is well recognized that the **CSF** provides a window into the presence of abnormal dementia proteins accumulating in the brain. CSF testing is a tool commonly used by neurologists for a range of conditions such as infection or brain inflammation. Some neurologic diagnoses such as these can only be made by sampling the CSF. In dementia, CSF has become a useful tool in detecting amyloid and tau, both of which are particularly relevant to Alzheimer's disease. CSF is obtained by a **lumbar puncture** (also known as a **spinal tap**), which can be performed in the office of many neurologic practices as an outpatient procedure. The lumbar puncture procedure is covered further in Appendix B. As is the case with nuclear medicine neuroimaging and for the same reasons detailed earlier, CSF analyses are currently limited in clinical practice to defining the differential diagnosis of dementia and are not used as a screening tool in people without symptoms. Other common forms of dementia, including dementia with Lewy bodies and frontotemporal dementia, lack definitive CSF biomarker patterns as seen in Alzheimer's disease.

> *Denise is a 68-year-old woman who has been experiencing 2 years of forgetfulness noticed by herself and others at work. Her parents died in their 50s from complications of smoking and heart attack. Nobody else in her family had memory problems with aging. She retired from work earlier than she had planned to focus on herself and her worsening memory problems. After seeing her primary care physician, she is referred to a neurologist specializing in dementia at a local academic center. Her history of increasing memory problems suggests Alzheimer's disease, but she begins to develop other features atypical for Alzheimer's disease, including tremor, slowness, and vivid dreams that she acts out. After a workup including bloodwork and MRI, she undergoes a lumbar puncture to clarify the diagnosis. After several weeks, CSF biomarker tests return and do not support the diagnosis of Alzheimer's disease. The neurologist reconsiders the diagnosis and, given the indications from the history and exam, as well as the CSF profile, makes a diagnosis of dementia with Lewy bodies instead. At age 75, Denise dies of pneumonia. Following her death, her family follows her wishes and donates her brain to research. At autopsy, the team finds prominent brain changes, including the presence of Lewy bodies, but very few Alzheimer's-type changes. For Denise, biomarker testing following lumbar puncture was the best way to make a diagnosis, above and beyond what the history, examination, and MRI revealed.*

Blood-based biomarkers

As noted earlier, both researchers in the dementia field and the public have considerable interest in the development of a blood-based test to diagnose dementia or even identify some forms of dementia before symptoms begin. Having a reliable blood test could make it much easier for dementia to be diagnosed early so that treatment could be started and responses tracked. Fortunately, a new era is beginning of blood-based biomarkers that can reliably identify very small circulating levels of brain proteins. Several biomarker blood tests for Alzheimer's disease are becoming available but may not be covered by insurance immediately. Their use is just now being appreciated, but they are expected to impact the diagnostic process, particularly given availability of newer treatments for Alzheimer's disease (Chapter 10).

Second opinions

It is important to feel confident that the correct approach to diagnosis and management has been taken. A second opinion can help in some cases, and most doctors are open to families pursuing one and may even encourage it.

Genetic testing

Sometimes families describe other people in their family who have had the same or a similar disorder. Although it may appear that an **inherited disorder** is being passed down through the generations, it may simply be that several older people in a family have developed dementia for unrelated or unknown reasons. For the most common forms of dementia such as Alzheimer's disease and frontotemporal dementia, less than half of families with a strong family history of dementia actually have an identifiable abnormal **gene** for dementia. Genes are codes within the **DNA** that tell cells in our body to make essential proteins that help our body run normally. Sometimes people are born with irregular, uncommon, or abnormal forms of genes that cause disease.

Several patterns of how genes are inherited from one generation to the next are shown in Table 2.1. In dementia, the most common genetic causes are either autosomal dominant or autosomal recessive.

TABLE 2.1 Genetic Inheritance Patterns

Inheritance pattern	Characteristics
Autosomal dominant	Each affected person usually has an affected parent; occurs in every generation in about half of those at risk
Autosomal recessive	Both parents of an affected person are carriers; not typically seen in every generation
X-linked dominant	Females are more frequently affected because all daughters and no sons of an affected man will be affected; can have affected males and females in same generation if the mother is affected
X-linked recessive	Males are more frequently affected; affected males often present in each generation
Maternal or mitochondrial	Can affect both males and females, but only passed on by females because all mitochondria of all children come from the mother; can appear in every generation

Adapted from: Genetic Alliance; The New York-Mid-Atlantic Consortium for Genetic and Newborn Screening Services. Understanding Genetics: A New York, Mid-Atlantic Guide for Patients and Health Professionals. Washington (DC): Genetic Alliance; 2009 Jul 8. APPENDIX E, INHERITANCE PATTERNS. Available from: https://www.ncbi.nlm.nih.gov/books/NBK115561/.

Genetic associations with dementia fall into two different categories: risk genes (or **alleles**) and deterministic genes. **Penetrance** is a genetic term describing how likely it is that a person will develop a disease when they have a gene, in this case dementia. Some genes increase the risk somewhat but have incomplete penetrance. Deterministic genes rarely occur but, when present, have nearly complete penetrance. With rare exception, if someone has one of those rare genes and lives long enough, they will develop dementia.

Alleles can be thought of as variations of a gene that everyone carries. Some genes have many variations, and some have only a handful. Everyone has two copies of most of the genes in DNA, which may be the same or different. As an example, let's consider an important gene often discussed in dementia called apolipoprotein E (*APOE*). *APOE* has three different versions called e2, e3, and e4 (these are often written with the Greek "ε" [epsilon], or ε2, ε3, or ε4). A person may carry two of these alleles in any combination, such as two e2s, two e4s, one e3 and one e4, and so forth. Depending on which mix of these two alleles someone has, the relative chances that they will develop dementia can be estimated. Carrying one or more e4s increases the risk of developing Alzheimer's disease (Chapter 5), and can be important in making decisions about some of the new treatments for Alzheimer's disease (Chapter 10).

However, several problems exist with testing for risk genes. First, they carry different risks in different populations—sometimes genes that are worrisome in some groups make no difference in others. Second, just because someone has the risky version of the genes does not mean that they will absolutely get dementia. Many people who have these risky genes live long lives without dementia, and many people who have no genetic factors get dementia early on. Third, currently, no changes in lifestyle or medications can be prescribed based on genetic profile alone.

In contrast, a second kind of gene acts very differently. Deterministic genes nearly always cause dementia or a related syndrome if the person lives long enough, and often dementia starts at a relatively young age. At least three deterministic genes are known in Alzheimer's disease, and at least six are associated with the spectrum of diseases in frontotemporal dementia. Testing for deterministic genes in dementia is done in select cases, typically in families with a strong family history of dementia in which about 50% of each generation (suggesting an autosomal dominant pattern) is affected by dementia or a related syndrome. The first person tested in a given family is ideally a patient with the disease to identify if the suspected gene is present in the first place. The presence of a given gene within that individual suggests a predictable risk of inheritance of that gene in other relatives. However, a negative or normal test does not exclude the chances of the same disorder appearing in other family members. This is because the test only checks for the specific gene being tested. Many families without an established genetic change have a familial pattern of dementia, but the exact genes that cause it are not yet known. Since these genes can appear out of the blue in some people with early-onset dementia, genetic testing may be suggested even if no family history is obvious.

Any decision to pursue genetic testing should be done with the input and knowledge of as many members of the family as possible or appropriate, as they will need to consider how to weigh the information relative to their own risk of disease. Such a discussion is ideally done under the careful supervision and assistance of a **genetic counselor**. It is very important to know that currently in the United States, people with genetic disorders are only legally protected against discrimination when it comes to health insurance. Although it may be tempting to seek out genetic information through commercially available direct-to-public marketing of genetic testing, knowledge of personal genetic information can adversely affect your ability to seek and obtain long-term care insurance and personal life and disability insurance policies, among others. Genetic information can be helpful, particularly as it may relate to actionable decisions, including life planning and fertility decisions (known as preimplantation genetic counseling). Through the coordinated efforts of specialists, **in** vitro fertilization (IVF) can prevent a known form of a gene, such as one that causes Alzheimer's disease, from being passed to the next generation.

Certainly, genetic testing is not for everyone for many reasons, including the psychological impact of knowing the genetic status of a family member. Although the dementia field has been patiently waiting for breakthroughs for years, it is hoped that more successful treatment options for **monogenetic**, or single-gene, causes of dementia and other diseases will be found in the near future. The current generation of family caregivers taking care of parents with genetically determined, often early-onset, dementia may very well see paradigm shifts in how we treat these diseases before they age into a period of increased risk for dementia.

CHAPTER 3

The Stages of Dementia

In this chapter, you will learn about:

- How the stages of dementia are determined
- The typical course of dementia, including how it may change in different stages of disease
- How to begin to anticipate changes in the course of dementia
- Why people with dementia die

People affected by dementia often want to have a better understanding of how dementia progresses, including why and when changes occur. It is only natural to want to know what the future holds from the early years of dementia to the end stages. It is also helpful to understand what lies ahead so that plans can be made for the future. Most forms of dementia are expected to worsen over time. The course of dementia differs from person to person, so anticipating exactly how and when changes occur is very challenging and usually not possible.

Staging dementia

Various names and stages are used for dementia progression. Some are descriptive, whereas others are numeric scales. Although they provide some general guidance, these names and stages usually lack the precision patients and families want in order to make plans. The course of Alzheimer's disease—its duration and the timing of changes—can be difficult to predict, and non-Alzheimer's dementias are even more challenging. People with dementia may pass through the following stages of mild, moderate, and severe dementia slowly or quickly:

- Mild, or early-stage, dementia: People with mild dementia may have recognizable and consistent cognitive problems that impact daily routines, but engagement often continues in simple social activities and lifelong hobbies. They often need help with coordinating medications, appointments, and daily schedules. Apathy and disengagement from regular life schedules may begin. They may begin to have problems with dexterity and coordination of movements.
- Moderate, or middle-stage, dementia: People with moderate dementia have a notable change in their ability to perform most activities of daily living, with greater reliance on others (Chapter 1). Symptoms of dementia become obvious to casual observers, and caregivers spend more time supporting basic needs such as hygiene and dressing. More obvious behavioral symptoms can emerge, including psychosis and aggression. Physical decline, including episodes of falling, is also apparent.
- Severe, or late-stage, dementia: People with severe dementia need caregiver support in nearly every aspect of care, including feeding, and communication and movement are often severely affected. They have limited mobility, are constantly confused, and eventually speak very little.

The exact duration of each stage can be difficult to predict, but a recognizable progression within each stage is nearly always seen, and when someone has moved from one stage to the next is apparent.

Prognosis: anticipating the future

The prognosis of dementia can be viewed in the short term (over the next few months) and the long term (what lies ahead further in the future). It is important to understand several points about prognosis:

- Absolute changes or discrete recent events often clarify the present needs but poorly predict the timing of future needs.
- The relative changes that occur over the course of a few months or a year can help anticipate the relative changes ahead over the same time frame.
- Looking back after 3 months, 6 months, or a year, a more rapid decline than was previously apparent may be recognized. Expectations can then be adjusted going forward.

With the exception of dementia immediately following a single large stroke and dementia resulting from untreated subcortical vascular disease (Chapter 7), all other forms of dementia progress over time. All degenerative forms of dementia progress, with noticeable changes from month to month and year to year. Sometimes patients experience an episode of delirium caused by infection or a change in medication, which may lead to new cognitive problems. Figure 3.1 demonstrates the typical relative changes in neurodegenerative dementias and dementia due to stroke.

Delving further into the patterns of progression, Figure 3.2 shows that a slow progression is generally seen in the early or mild stages of disease, followed by a more rapid and noticeable set of changes in the moderate stage when functional independence is lost. In the later severe stages of dementia, some people with dementia remain physically active and mobile, with slowly evolving cognitive changes over time. For others, especially those affected by parkinsonism (such as is seen in dementia with Lewy bodies [DLB]), variability may exist within the stages, especially in mild to moderate disease. Superimposed non-neurologic physical problems, such as frailty or arthritis, can make falls more likely and further influence the course. As persons near late-stage or severe dementia, physical function and swallowing are increasingly affected, and people with advanced dementia become

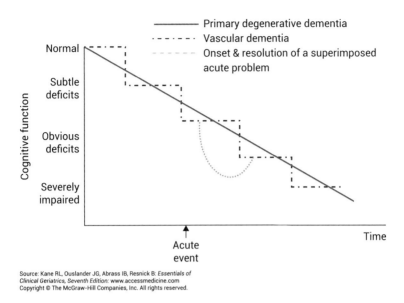

FIGURE 3.1 **Patterns of progression in dementia over time.** Progression in
dementia depends on the underlying cause. In the most common forms, such
as Alzheimer's disease and frontotemporal dementia, progression is gradual
but becomes more obvious and severe over time. Stroke may cause sudden
or stepwise decline, and sometimes modest recovery occurs after each stroke.
Dementia with Lewy bodies is notable for spontaneous fluctuations but with an
underlying progression over time.

dependent on others for nearly everything. Overall, more than two-
thirds of functional abilities are lost in the final stage of dementia,
which is known as the **terminal decline**.

Rapidly progressive dementias, such as Creutzfeldt–Jakob disease,
tend to show rapid symptomatic changes even by the day or week.
The symptoms that appear first (e.g., memory problems) will typically become more profound over time. Behavioral changes such as
agitation may emerge, particularly in the moderate stage when hyper-
active behaviors emerge (Chapters 1 and 2). Conversely, for some
people, obsessive personality features in frontotemporal dementia or
hallucinations in dementia with Lewy bodies may recede with disease

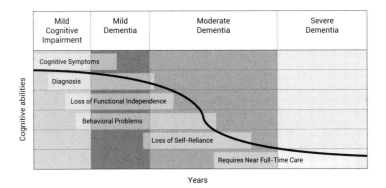

FIGURE 3.2 **Progression from mild cognitive impairment to severe dementia.** Taking a closer look at progression, even gradually progressive diseases have changes in the tempo of disease over time. Shown here is the typical progression seen in Alzheimer's disease. Changes are slow at the beginning, faster in the middle stages, and again slower or less obvious in later stages of the disease.

progression. These and other behavioral symptoms may emerge at unexpected times or recur briefly at unexpected intervals. Generally, most people become quieter, more docile, more confused, and less mobile over time.

Life expectancy in dementia

The average life expectancy in Alzheimer's disease from time of diagnosis to death is about 5 years, although some may have a much shorter course (as short as 2 years from first symptoms) and others have a much longer course (as long as 20 years). This wide range of longevity underscores some of the mystery of the disease and the marked variability of its presentation. These numbers are based on community-based studies in which the timing of the disease onset was identified through intense screening programs. In contrast, life expectancy in other forms of dementia (non-Alzheimer's) is not well understood, and many people live with dementia for years before seeing a doctor and receiving a diagnosis. People with frontotemporal dementia may live longer than some people with Alzheimer's disease, although their longevity may be substantially foreshortened if weakness due to frontotemporal dementia–associated amyotrophic lateral sclerosis develops. Knowledge of the average life expectancy in dementia with Lewy bodies is limited but is thought to be similar to Alzheimer's disease. Rarely, persons with dementia with Lewy bodies may develop rapid eye movement (REM) sleep behavior disorder 20 to 30 years before the first cognitive symptoms are seen. In most dementias, it is understood that most microscopic brain changes begin 10 to 15 years before the first cognitive symptoms begin (Chapter 2).

Why does someone with dementia die?

Most often, dementia does not cause death shortly after diagnosis, and most people with dementia die in their 60s or later. The age at death often depends on the age when symptoms began, the general underlying health of the person with dementia, and the support to which they have access, especially in later stages. Most forms of dementia progress slowly, and patients in later stages also progress slowly unless they experience a catastrophic event, such as a fall or a complication from a medical illness. Most people with dementia who gradually progress into a severe stage develop complications from immobility and begin to experience problems from becoming bedbound or coordinating chewing and swallowing. Once a patient becomes bedbound, **decubitus ulcers** (bedsores), skin infections, and blood clots in the legs and lungs can develop and urinary tract infections become common. When a person with dementia loses the ability to coordinate chewing and swallowing, it can lead to problems with maintaining nutrition and **aspiration pneumonia** (a type of lung infection) can occur when food or even saliva is accidentally inhaled rather than swallowed.

A general understanding of the stages of dementia will help with planning for the future, also known as advance care planning, which is discussed in Chapter 15. The stages of dementia also lead to important changes in the needs of people affected by dementia, a subject further covered in Chapters 13 and 14.

CHAPTER 4

Where, Why, and How Dementia Affects the Brain

In this chapter, you will learn about:

- How the nervous system is organized and its primary functions
- The relevant anatomy and how it changes in dementia
- The main cells of the nervous system

U nderstanding how the brain works can sometimes help us face the problems caused by dementia in each of its stages. This chapter discusses brain anatomy from its structure to its microscopic cells, how the parts of the brain relate to one another, how dementia develops, and why certain symptoms occur.

Substantial advances in knowledge of how the brain works have occurred in the past century, particularly in the past 2 decades. The field has moved from understanding how the brain works by observing changes after injury to gaining a better understanding through studying healthy people using complex brain imaging. What has become clear is that the brain is constantly in flux, with billions of active brain circuits constantly being activated or blocked, speeded up or slowed down. Even an aging brain can create new cells and new connections.

The nervous system and its structure: from the big picture to the small cells

The human body has three nervous systems. The **central nervous system** includes the brain and related structures in the head along with the spinal cord. The **peripheral nervous system** is made up of all of the nerves that exit the brain and spinal cord; it carries sensory information from the skin and body and sends movement signals from the spinal cord to muscles in the arms, legs, and trunk. The third nervous system combines parts of the central and peripheral nervous systems and is called the **autonomic nervous system**. The autonomic nervous system is often known for the "fight or flight" reaction, but it does much more than protect us in potentially harmful situations. It also helps to regulate and control blood pressure and heart rate, body temperature, urination, bowel movements, and sexual function.

The brain is the biggest structure in the central nervous system. The main part of the brain is called the **cerebrum**, also known as the **cerebral cortex**, which is the part of the brain responsible for memory, thinking, perception, and behavior and for making body movements in smooth coordinated ways. The cerebrum is organized into four main regions or lobes, **frontal, parietal, temporal, and occipital**, each with a different job (Figure 4.1). Each side of the brain contains its own four lobes that together are known as a brain's **hemisphere**. In addition, a main area deeper in the brain called the **cerebellum** and a series of structures collectively called the **brainstem** have important functions related to movement, coordination, and balance, but these areas also affect thinking and memory.

The **spinal cord** is the other major structure that makes up the central nervous system. The spinal cord serves as a highway connecting sensations from the body to the brain. Signals traveling from the brain to the body make the limbs move, passing from the central nervous system to the peripheral nervous system. From there, the peripheral nerves project to muscles to create movement, and other nerves transmit sensory information back to the central nervous system. The spinal cord and peripheral nervous system connect to form an important reflex arc so that when you touch a hot stove, your arm reflexively and instantaneously jerks away.

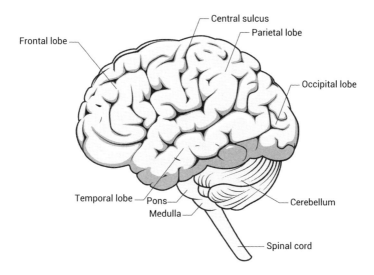

FIGURE 4.1 **The brain: lobes, cerebellum, and brainstem.** The main parts, or lobes, of the brain are involved in all forms of dementia. The brainstem connects the brain to the rest of the nervous system and becomes the spinal cord lower down.

Also important to understand is that the brain is organized in a highly complex manner; in most people, each side of the brain has different responsibilities, all contributing to the whole of brain function. For everyone, the side of the brain responsible for language is called the dominant side. The left side of the brain is dominant in most people, in about 9 out of 10 right-handed people and around half of left-handed people. The side of brain dominance can have implications in how dementia may present, especially if a focal process, such as a tumor or stroke, affects the dominant (mostly likely left) side of the brain.

The lobes of the brain

To best understand the process of dementia, it is important to understand the lobes of the cerebrum (frontal, parietal, temporal, and occipital) and their functions (Figure 4.1). Each lobe has great importance in life, and each has distinct functions that may demonstrate problems when affected by dementia.

Frontal lobes

The frontal lobes have many functions, including generation of abstract thought, complex reasoning, and movement. This area of the brain is responsible for coming up with an idea, understanding a proverb, or slogging through a tough book. It helps us shift between one set of ideas and another (so-called multitasking), planning a series of events (considering a day's schedule or working on a home repair), or accomplishing a single physical task or a sequence of tasks we know well (riding a bicycle, signing one's name, or putting on a necktie). The frontal lobes are also thought to be the areas responsible for personality traits and behavior and how we interact, engage, and respond to one another with appropriate emotional responses. Other frontal lobe regions are responsible for keeping us in a relatively well-balanced mood. The dominant frontal lobe is responsible for generating fluent speech. In dementia and disabling psychiatric disorders, when the frontal lobe is involved, behavioral or mood changes such as depression, obsessive-compulsive features, or excessive anxiety are often observed. This may cause the personality to change, affecting social interactions and relationships.

Temporal lobes

Like the frontal lobes, each of the two temporal lobes has a number of functions, and they include a key structure for memory called the **hippocampus** (plural, hippocampi). The earliest microscopic changes causing memory loss in Alzheimer's disease often begin in the hippocampi and their networks. In a left brain–dominant person, the left hippocampus is principally responsible for **verbal memory** (learning a story or a list of unrelated words), whereas the right hippocampus is principally responsible for **visuospatial memory** (remembering a planned path or series of intended directions). The primary role of the hippocampi and their circuitry is to transition newly acquired information into long-term memory. In contrast, **crystallized knowledge**—someone's personal, established knowledge learned through formal education and autobiographical experiences across a lifespan—is more broadly represented throughout the brain.

As is the case with the frontal lobes, one of the temporal lobes is principally involved with language function (typically the left temporal lobe). When the temporal lobe responsible for language is impaired, someone may inappropriately respond to questions or directions and may speak in a way that sounds jumbled. Early on, some people may search for words and simplify what they say. They seem like they have the word just on the tip of their tongue but they can't quite find it, or eventually they may say something like, "What's that thing where you put the cold beer and milk and the eggs? Oh yes, the refrigerator." Or some may say nearly correct words: "I need a knife for my soup" or "I need a spoon for my sloop"; these are called **paraphasias**. Others may include unrelated information in their speech, such as brief non sequiturs (e.g., "When you saw me at the pool last week . . . ready for dinner now"), or even include nonsensical word-like sounds (**neologisms**) in a jumbled "**word salad**," for example "footfall, time, it on, last week, frownt").

Occipital lobes

The occipital lobes are principally responsible for vision, with one occipital lobe perceiving the opposite side of the world in its visual field. When the occipital lobe is affected by dementia or stroke, a complex change in vision or the loss of part of the visual field altogether may occur. Patients may sometimes have misperceptions, including distorted colors, sizes, or shapes, or misperceptions about the positions of objects nearby. **Visual hallucinations** (spontaneously occurring, often complex images) are thought to arise from the occipital lobe. The visual hallucinations common in dementia with Lewy bodies are usually of people, small animals, or insects. Primary vision loss (due to cataracts or diseases of the eye) can further complicate visual misperceptions.

Parietal lobes

The parietal cortex is one of the most complex regions of the brain and the hardest to understand and explain. At its simplest, it is a sensory and information integration center, combining visual, language, sensory, and motor information from other parts of the brain to provide a sense of self, including body image, limb position, and direction of movement of the person as well as relation to objects within the environment or the environment itself around the person. It also connects information about what someone sees with the information the brain can connect with the image. The parietal cortex is often affected in Alzheimer's disease and is associated with changes in language and with the ability to recognize familiar surroundings or how to get from one well-known place to another. Driving abilities may be particularly sensitive to changes in parietal lobe function since complex visuospatial skills are needed to perceive the position of the car in a moving environment.

Deeper brain structures

Deep within the brain are other important structures, but these are mostly associated with body movement. Nonetheless, they can have implications for cognition and memory and are particularly important in people who have slowness and stiffness in addition to dementia, more broadly described as parkinsonism (Chapters 5 and 6). These deep structures are broadly called the **basal ganglia** and include the caudate nucleus and globus pallidus. The caudate nucleus is the main site of pathologic changes in Huntington's disease and leads to abnormal irregular movements called chorea.

Connecting the brain, basal ganglia, and cerebellum to the spinal cord is the brainstem, which is made up of an uppermost part (the midbrain) and two lower regions (the pons and medulla) (Figure 4.1). These are relatively small structures and serve to deliver electrical signals through the spinal cord to the arms and legs for sensation and movement. The main brain changes in Parkinson's disease occur in the basal ganglia circuits, which are connected to a small region in the midbrain. The brainstem is also essential for the movement and sensation of the eyes, face, and throat. One possible cause of dementia, called **progressive supranuclear palsy** (PSP), can affect eye movements. PSP is associated with atrophy (shrinkage) and microscopic changes in the midbrain (PSP is covered further in Chapter 7). In nearly all forms of late-stage dementia, swallowing can be affected. This relates to pathologic changes in the lower brainstem along with centers and automatic pathways coordinating swallowing in the cortex and basal ganglia.

The vascular supply of the brain

Feeding the brain is a network of **blood vessels** that branch off the **aorta** (the large artery that comes directly off the heart) through the **carotid arteries** (in the neck) to supply the front parts of the brain and the **vertebral arteries** (also in the neck) to supply the back parts of the brain. These vessels all reconnect in a loop at the base of the brain to allow for a consistent blood supply for the high-energy brain. A blockage or disruption of blood flow through any of the brain's many blood vessels causes **stroke**. When some of the bigger vessels are blocked in stroke, large regions of the brain (such as the cerebellum or brainstem) may be affected and unable to function normally. Although dementia is typically thought of as being a gradual process, in stroke, brain regions are suddenly unable to function and may cause cognitive or motoric problems similar to those seen in other forms of dementia.

As the vessels pass into the brain they get smaller and smaller, down to the **capillary**, which is just big enough to carry a few oxygen-rich red blood cells. At this point, nutrients and oxygen are extracted across the blood vessel wall and into the **astrocytes** and then passed into the brain, including the **neurons**. A key feature of the nervous system is a tight barrier between the capillaries and the brain called the **blood–brain barrier**, which limits toxins, germs, and even some medications from entering the brain. The coupling of the blood vessel to a neuron and its surrounding cells and microenvironment is called the **neurovascular unit**. It is also at this point where byproducts of brain metabolism are passed back into the blood to be sent back to the heart and cleaned by the liver and kidneys, with oxygen getting replenished through the lungs.

Microscopic view of the brain

The cells that make up the brain fall into two broad categories: neurons (nerve cells) and **glia** (everything else) (Figure 4.2). Neurons are the cells that generate and communicate electrical signals to other nerve cells. Glia serve to support neurons both physically and functionally. Glia include several types of cells, including **oligodendrocytes** (which make up the **white matter** that insulates the electrical connections), astrocytes (which provide nutrients to the cells), **ependymal cells** (which create the border around the fluid-filled spaces called ventricles), and **microglia** (immune cells in the brain that fight infection and control inflammation). All these cell types are located

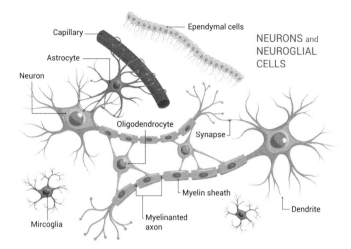

FIGURE 4.2 **Cells and microscopic structures of the central nervous system.** Nerve cells (or neurons) are the primary cells that generate electrical activity in the brain. They are fed nutrients through the small vessels (capillaries) and supported by astrocytes and protected by microglia. Neurons connect with one another through long axon projections that are insulated by myelin made by oligodendrocytes. Injury to any one of these cells, either in one spot or many, can impact the brain and cause neurologic symptoms.

throughout the brain and the rest of the central nervous system. Neurons are primarily located in the outer rim of the brain, known as the **gray matter,** surrounded by astrocytes and microglia. Neurons are also present in the basal ganglia, brainstem, and spinal cord, but they are not as closely related to cognition. The long connections of neurons (called **axons**) pass through the deeper areas of the brain known as the white matter.

How microscopic changes occur in each specific form of dementia (Table 1.1) is discussed in the next few chapters. Overall, it is important to understand that the anatomy of the brain is complex and that a complex set of changes at the microscopic level affects the brain of people with dementia, leading to changes in how multiple brain regions function and interact and thus causing dementia symptoms.

Cerebrospinal fluid

Cerebrospinal fluid (CSF) is a clear, colorless, naturally occurring fluid created by structures within the brain called the **choroid plexus**. From the choroid plexus, CSF goes directly into the ventricular system of the brain and circulates around the brain and down around the spinal cord into the lower back. As this fluid circulates, it is resorbed at the top of the brain (vertex) through small structures called **arachnoid granulations**. In recent years, understanding of the function of CSF has shifted from a fluid that largely serves as a cushion for the brain to that of a system with important roles in the clearance and movement of various substances out of the brain. As discussed in Chapter 2, testing brain-based biomarker proteins in the CSF has become a helpful tool in determining whether dementia is due to Alzheimer's disease or a related cause.

The relationship between brain anatomy and brain changes in dementia

Brain cells located throughout the brain are in, many ways, indistinguishable from one another. They are organized in layers and connect with one another or support the brain's metabolism. Yet for reasons not entirely understood, brain changes in dementia begin in certain brain regions and appear in nearby areas. Research suggests some changes in dementia occur across a network of related brain circuits, but how this occurs is uncertain. It may also be that some regions of nerve cells are vulnerable to changes and injury over time in ways not fully understood.

Underlying the most common causes of progressive dementia are two main concepts: **protein aggregation** and **neurodegeneration**. Although dementias can differ substantially clinically, they can overlap **neuropathologically** (the changes that can be seen under the microscope). In nearly all forms of neurodegeneration, which causes most forms of dementia, a common finding of some form of an abnormal protein that has begun to aggregate and become toxic to the brain is seen. Then through a cascade of events, the process of neurodegeneration begins. Neurodegeneration describes brain cells that gradually become sick, wither, and die. It may be that neurodegeneration occurs simultaneously in many brain cells related to one another throughout the brain or that a connected network of cells may become diseased one by one, side by side, on a grand scale. This remains a matter of intense research. The specific forms of dementia and how they vary substantially in their underlying cellular brain changes (also known as the disease **pathophysiology**) are discussed in later chapters.

In most forms of dementia, one or more **proteins** begin to misfold and gather (or aggregate) in the brain for reasons that are not entirely understood and in a way that can't yet be controlled or slowed down. It is likely that these protein aggregates are toxic to brain cells, or it could be that these aggregates are just signs that something toxic is happening to the brain cells that leads to neurodegeneration. But a lot of progress has been made in recent years, including shifts in how we think about why brain changes in dementia happen. Failed research trials have led to new thinking and hope for new discoveries.

Three of the main brain proteins being studied in dementia are **amyloid** (also known as amyloid-beta), **tau**, and **synuclein** (also known as α-**synuclein**). Many other brain proteins are of interest to researchers, but these are the three seen over and again in dementia. (To be clear, these proteins have nothing to do with what you eat. There are proteins in food, and there are proteins found throughout our body, including the brain, but they are not directly related.) These three proteins have a normal function and exist throughout the brain and even elsewhere in the body. For complicated reasons not fully understood, in neurodegenerative dementias, these proteins begin to fold and clump or **aggregate** in ways that become toxic to normal brain cell metabolism and function. In Alzheimer's disease, the two main proteins involved are tau (which aggregates mostly inside the cell) and amyloid (which aggregates outside the cell); this is reviewed further in Chapter 5. Some other forms of dementia are thought to be primarily due to protein becoming aggregated.

In addition to the three main proteins found in the most common types of dementia (amyloid, tau, and synuclein), other proteins, including **TDP-43** and **prion**, are important in some less common forms of dementia. TDP-43 has also been recently found to be present in a high number of patients with clinical symptoms of Alzheimer's disease.

Understanding how these proteins differ is important scientifically as breakthrough treatments are sought to target amyloid and tau in Alzheimer's disease, synuclein in dementia with Lewy bodies and Parkinson's disease, tau and TDP-43 in the frontotemporal dementias, and a prion protein in **Creutzfeldt–Jakob disease**. Sometimes several types of protein aggregates are seen in a single person with dementia.

Neurotransmission: how nerve cells talk to one another

Communication and signaling between normal brain cells take place through the exchange of small proteins called **neurotransmitters** (Figure 4.3). These neurotransmitters are released when an electrical signal created by one brain cell is received by the next cell. Most medications used in treating dementia interact with neurotransmitters, either blocking them or making them last longer once released from nerve cells. In most forms of dementia, protein aggregation begins to impact the intensity of neurotransmission from one nerve cell to the next. Take any one of these proteins (e.g., amyloid or tau) and imagine that it is accumulating in and around two cells in the brain that routinely communicate with one another. Even as brain cells weaken and begin to die from these neurodegenerative changes, these two

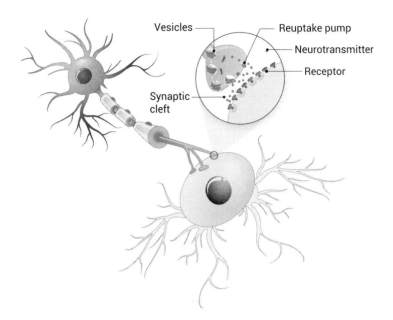

FIGURE 4.3 **Neurotransmitters in the nervous system.** Neurotransmitters are small natural chemicals that trigger an electrical signal activating or suppressing the function of nerve cells as they communicate with one another. Most currently available medications used in treating dementia interact with neurotransmitters.

cells continue to talk to one another but less and less over time as the changes progress. Now imagine that this process of communication (and neurodegeneration) is taking place on billions of nerve cells, all of which communicate with numerous other nerve cells side by side and in a network connecting with other more distant nerve cells. These neurodegenerative changes and how they impact the person with dementia are fundamental to the most common forms of dementia.

Complicating matters further, about one-third of people in their 70s and 80s will have microscopic evidence of protein aggregation and neurodegeneration but no clinical evidence of cognitive impairment.

For example, when we look at the brains of two people with neuropathologic Alzheimer's changes, the person who has symptoms such as memory loss and the person who does not cannot always be predicted. Thus, while the microscopic changes of dementia are important, they are not the entire story.

Most of the medications available to treat dementia either increase the amount of neurotransmitter released or allow the neurotransmitter to remain for a longer period of time, with a net effect of strengthening cell-to-cell communication. But because the cells at either end of this connection continue to weaken, the signs and symptoms of dementia continue to progress. In scientific research, several greatly debated questions remain, including whether these abnormal proteins cause dementia or are simply evidence of dementia. Most medications being tried in research studies for dementia attempt to remove these proteins or stop them from accumulating in the first place. We are just starting to enter a fundamentally new phase of dementia care in which new treatments target the biological changes of disease, and hopefully begin to make long-term impacts on microscopic brain changes.

The next few chapters use what you learned in this chapter to help you understand the changes in the most common forms of dementia and how medications used for dementia work, beginning with the most common causes of dementia due to neurodegenerative changes (Alzheimer's disease, dementia with Lewy bodies, and frontotemporal dementia), followed by stroke and other less common causes of dementia. Later chapters discuss treatment options, practical tools to manage dementia, care for the caregiver, and research throughout the course of dementia.

CHAPTER 5

Alzheimer's Disease

In this chapter, you will learn about:

- The key signs and symptoms leading to a diagnosis of Alzheimer's disease
- Alzheimer's disease when it presents with or without memory loss
- Changes in behavior, mood, and sleep in Alzheimer's disease
- Balance and movement problems in Alzheimer's disease
- What causes Alzheimer's disease
- How Alzheimer's disease is diagnosed

Alzheimer's disease is the most common cause of dementia, representing at least 70% of all persons with dementia and affecting approximately 15% of all people over 65 years of age, making it the most common neurologic disorder in this age group and one of the most common medical disorders associated with aging. For unclear reasons, it affects women more than men. Some studies suggest that nearly half of all people over the age of 85 have some evidence of Alzheimer's-type changes. It is thought that approximately 80% of nursing home residents are admitted because of advancing Alzheimer's disease.

Alzheimer's disease is named for Dr. Alois Alzheimer, a German neurologist who first described the disease in 1901. He noted the main changes in the brain, beginning with shrinkage or atrophy of some regions of the brain, particularly in those we now know are important for memory (Figure 2.1). Dr. Alzheimer also first described, and even drew, the microscopic changes of the disease that are still recognized and studied today: plaques (largely made up of aggregated amyloid) and tangles (dying nerve cells filled with aggregated tau). These changes, which are toxic to brain cells and neurotransmitters (Chapter 4), are shown in further detail in Figure 5.1. Until the 1970s, Alzheimer's disease was considered just a "presenile" dementia. It was once thought that everyone who lived long enough would develop dementia and that dementia was part of the normal aging process. Following the rise in life expectancy over the last half of the 20th century, greater numbers of people began living into their 80s, 90s, and beyond. With this aging population, more people developed dementia, but also many people aged without dementia, leading to new concepts about normal aging versus pathologic brain changes.

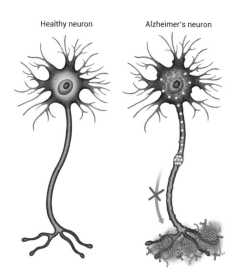

FIGURE 5.1 How Alzheimer's disease affects neurons (nerve cells). Neuritic plaques (which include clumped amyloid protein) and tau aggregates (which clump in the neuron itself and are called tangles) are two microscopic changes seen in Alzheimer's disease. The complex triggers leading to each of these changes are the targets of intense investigations looking for new treatments.

As reviewed in Chapter 4, the microscopic brain changes in Alzheimer's disease are caused by the clumping of two proteins, amyloid and tau, in certain regions of the brain. Many different factors likely contribute to these brain changes. The brain regions involved usually determine the symptoms that are seen. But why these two normal brain proteins begin to clump in some people as they age and not in everyone remains uncertain. In Alzheimer's disease, amyloid plaques may be the first obvious changes for most people, followed by tau-filled tangles (also known as neurofibrillary tangles). It is thought that symptom onset and progression closely follow the development of tangles.

Signs and symptoms of Alzheimer's disease

Memory loss is most often recognized as the earliest or most significant symptom over the course of Alzheimer's disease. This amnestic form of Alzheimer's disease (related to **amnesia**, referring to Alzheimer's disease with memory loss) is seen in approximately three out of four people who have Alzheimer's disease. Three other nonamnestic presentations are less common as the initial or primary symptoms: the **frontal-executive**, language, and **visuospatial presentations** of Alzheimer's disease. Eventually all types of symptoms are seen in nearly all people by late stage Alzheimer's disease.

Memory loss in Alzheimer's disease can begin initially with seemingly ordinary lapses in memory, such as misplacing objects (e.g., keys, wallet, glasses), but becomes more serious when items are permanently lost and need replacement. Repetition in conversation (telling stories over and over or asking the same questions repeatedly) is common and can be distressing, especially if caregivers need to repeat themselves often. Inattention to bills, appointments, and taking medications may also be symptoms of forgetfulness. Forgetfulness may be characterized by greater reliance on calendars, lists, and reminder notes as well as by getting lost in local familiar neighborhoods.

Rhoda is an 81-year-old woman whose husband has noticed her increasing forgetfulness over the past 2 years. At first, she began misplacing objects at home, but she recently had to replace her wallet and its contents after it could not be located. Friends notice she increasingly repeats the same questions at dinner, and she recently got lost while driving in her neighborhood. Her husband brings these concerns to the attention of their primary care physician, who finds that Rhoda cannot recall the date and has difficulty remembering information they just discussed. Testing, including bloodwork and a brain MRI, shows only mild brain atrophy in the temporal lobes, especially the hippocampi. Alzheimer's disease is diagnosed, and a treatment plan is coordinated with her husband.

Rhoda's story is typical of the amnestic form of Alzheimer's disease. Memory loss is not the only symptom in Alzheimer's disease, and some people with Alzheimer's have very different problems, including visuospatial impairment (getting lost or confused in familiar environments). Sometimes it can be difficult to tell when someone does not recognize where they are, or have just forgotten how they got there, and sometimes these symptoms can occur together. When Alzheimer's disease changes occur only or primarily in the rear parts of the brain, including the occipital and parietal lobes, it is called **posterior cortical atrophy**. Other forms of Alzheimer's disease include one with primary language decline (particularly word-finding difficulty, known as **logopenia** or **logopenic primary progressive aphasia**) and one with personality changes and frontal-executive dysfunction, called the frontal-executive form. Most often, hints of each of these problems are seen in people who first or primarily have noticeable memory problems. Alzheimer's disease that presents with more physically obvious changes is called **corticobasal syndrome**, in which **parkinsonian** motor symptoms (stiffness, slowness, rigidity, and/or tremor) may be noticeable on one side of the body or both. The physical changes in Alzheimer's disease, including **parkinsonism**, are reviewed later in this chapter. People with corticobasal syndrome can also have changes in language and visuospatial abilities.

Roberto, a 73-year-old man, spent the last 40 years repairing and restoring vintage American cars. He continues to drive well, hasn't gotten lost, and can troubleshoot mechanical car problems better than anyone else in their family business. Three years ago, his son (and partner in their car restoration business) began noticing that his father was having difficulty naming common tools in the garage. His father either needed to describe the object in several phrases or recalled it only in Spanish, his primary language from childhood. Over the past year, Roberto's language decline has become much more apparent. His wife has to help him complete his sentences or, worse yet, goes through a series of yes/no questions to get his thoughts expressed correctly. Testing, including cerebrospinal fluid biomarkers, shows Roberto has the language (logopenic) form of Alzheimer's disease. As time goes on, his language and memory worsen.

As reviewed here, many different forms of dementia have come to be called "Alzheimer's disease" because Alzheimer's-type changes are found in the brain in all these forms. The type of symptoms is determined by where the microscopic brain changes of aggregation and neurodegeneration occur. Individual differences are seen in how the disease presents from person to person. To review the workup for dementia and how Alzheimer's is specifically diagnosed, turn back to Chapter 2.

Take-home point

All people with Alzheimer's disease have a slowly progressive brain disorder that affects memory, thinking, behavior, and movement, but they may differ in the rate of change and severity of the disease.

Behavioral and psychological symptoms of Alzheimer's disease

In addition to cognitive problems such as memory loss or language impairment, Alzheimer's disease frequently presents with a group of mood symptoms collectively termed **behavioral and psychological symptoms of dementia** or **neuropsychiatric symptoms** of dementia. Symptoms can range from apathy and depression to anxiety, anger, irritability, and aggression, and even to profound hallucinations and delusions, with the most disruptive and disabling symptoms accompanying worsening disease stages. Behavioral and psychological symptoms of dementia can be very difficult to predict; they may not occur at all, may occur to a mild and manageable degree, or may occur with more severity over a long period of time. This section describes these symptoms; treatment of the symptoms is discussed in Chapter 11.

Apathy, depression, and anhedonia

Apathy (losing interest in doing things) is a prominent expression of behavioral and psychological symptoms of dementia in Alzheimer's disease. Apathy is closely related to **anhedonia** (or a lack of pleasure); in Alzheimer's disease, both apathy and anhedonia lead to a lack of initiative or inertia in doing things. Although depression is a term used to describe mood symptoms in Alzheimer's disease and may have been diagnosed before Alzheimer's disease, true depression in Alzheimer's disease is uncommon. Depression refers to episodes of "the blues," with sadness, despair, tearfulness, and, in some cases, apathy. Apathy in people with Alzheimer's disease can be an early subtle symptom in which they seem unexpectedly content when idle and previously enjoyed hobbies are neglected. Apathy in Alzheimer's disease can be particularly stubborn and persistent. Few, if any, medications are effective in treating it, although medications used in depression may be tried.

Sally's husband reports that his wife has been increasingly for-getful over the past year. Six months ago, she needed reminders to complete plans for a party for her 72nd birthday. Three months ago, she made several errors in well-known family recipes that she prepared for a potluck. Sally had been an avid participant in a local choral group, but about 2 years ago she inexplicably stopped going to rehearsals, which she initially attributed to a falling out with others in the group. Over the past few weeks, she has awak-ened several times in the middle of the night to prepare to go to work and became upset with her husband when he tried to get her to return to bed.

As his concerns grow, Sally's husband convinces her to see her physician. A neurologic examination reveals she has difficulty stating the day of the week and cannot remember a list of three words she had read back to her physician just 5 minutes ear-lier. Throughout the examination, she interrupts the physician to protest the need for her visit, indicating that her memory was completely normal. A review of basic laboratory and imaging tests does not reveal any metabolic abnormality or alterna-tive cause for what is most likely the early stage of Alzheimer's disease.

Delusions

Some behavioral disruptions in Alzheimer's disease can come to define the illness for patients and their families. **Delusions** (fixed false beliefs) are common but are not part of the course of disease for all people. However, they can be particularly noticeable, upset-ting, or persistent, depending on the content. Delusions can be rela-tively innocuous if they are only noticeable now and then, last for just minutes, and don't lead to disagreements, but they can become disruptive when they are more frequent or have a threatening quality.

Delusions may occur because of the brain's effort to fill in missing gaps in knowledge with a reasonable explanation. For example, in the course of normal adult life, if a wallet is lost, a reasonable cause would be theft. However, a person with Alzheimer's disease who loses a wallet at a store counter might call someone else a thief, although there was no theft. When a disconnect exists between reality and beliefs—something is highly unlikely but strongly believed—it is a delusion. Sometimes delusions can lead to episodes and cycles of irritability and anger, especially when they are intensely believed by the person affected by Alzheimer's disease.

Agitation and aggression

Delusions may be accompanied by a heightened stress response called **agitation**. Agitation describes nervous excitement, sometimes accompanied by pacing, impatience, or a short temper. Heightened levels of agitation can lead to **aggression**, with shouting or even physically aggressive behaviors such as punching or kicking, even at loved ones. Delusions with agitation can occur at unexpected times but sometimes may be predictable, such as after a night without sleep or when traveling and being in an unfamiliar place at bedtime. Agitation may develop when memory lapses are challenged, especially when the person does not recognize they have memory problems. Periods of confusion and agitation that tend to occur late in the day are called **sundowning**.

Sleep

Sleep patterns often change in Alzheimer's disease. The stages of sleep may be very disorganized or occur in rapid cycles, and some people may lack periods of deep restorative sleep altogether. In the early to middle stages of the disease, fragmented sleep and insomnia can be strong determinants of quality of life for caregivers. Sleep patterns of caregivers become equally disrupted, and patience can become strained. Although insomnia is common, so is excessive daytime fatigue.

Changes in movement and balance in Alzheimer's disease

About 1 in 6 people with Alzheimer's disease has mild problems with stiffness and slowness of arm or body movements and may even have tremor or limb shakiness at the time of diagnosis. Changes in how the body moves become increasingly common in the later stages of disease and can have important implications for care, which are reviewed in Chapters 13 and 14. These physical changes are termed **parkinsonism**; parkinsonism describes a group of motor symptoms, including stiffness, slowness, walking difficulty, imbalance, and tremor. In contrast to Parkinson's disease, memory difficulties are the main problems in Alzheimer's disease and the motor difficulties are milder.

As we age, the risk of developing more than one neurologic problem increases, and some people with Parkinson's disease may also develop Alzheimer's disease and vice versa. Why two disorders occur in the same person is unclear; no definite connection has been identified other than age being a risk factor for both Alzheimer's disease and Parkinson's disease. Parkinson's disease and Parkinson's disease dementia are discussed in Chapter 6.

What causes Alzheimer's disease?

Several biological pathways lead to metabolic and microscopic changes in Alzheimer's disease. Why they occur remains a mystery and may relate to certain risk factors. The strongest risk factors for developing Alzheimer's disease include advancing age, low childhood education, and vascular diseases such as stroke and cardiovascular disease. Other established risk factors for Alzheimer's disease include **diabetes**, midlife obesity and midlife **hypertension**, smoking, a sedentary lifestyle, and a diet unhealthy for the heart. All these risk factors are further influenced by our genetics. Women may have a higher risk for developing Alzheimer's disease, but this may be an artifact of differences in life expectancy. It is generally a good idea to address and avoid any reversible risk factors, but the value of doing so remains uncertain. Even taking all these risk factors into consideration, about half of all people who develop Alzheimer's disease have no known risk factors other than increasing age.

In recent years, the genetics of Alzheimer's disease have influenced thinking about how Alzheimer's disease occurs. Although rare, strong family histories of early-onset Alzheimer's disease are associated with a few known deterministic genes: presenilin 1 (*PSEN1*), presenilin 2 (*PSEN2*), and amyloid precursor protein (*APP*). Although genetic testing for the nearly three dozen alleles for late-onset Alzheimer's disease risk is generally not recommended (Chapter 2), these genes have identified a few key pathways and provided new insight into the disease. Wide variation is seen in how common these genes are in the population and how likely they are to cause Alzheimer's disease (Figure 5.2). Studying genes and how they work has led in several new directions that have helped us move beyond traditional ways of thinking about Alzheimer's disease. These include a new appreciation for how the immune system impacts Alzheimer's disease and an awareness of how Alzheimer's may develop when the movement of proteins and fluids in and around brain cells gets interrupted.

Diagnostic testing for Alzheimer's disease

As detailed in Chapter 2, diagnosing Alzheimer's disease begins with a doctor taking a history and performing a complete

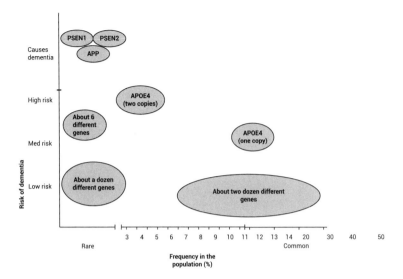

FIGURE 5.2 **Genetic variants and risk of Alzheimer's disease.** More than three dozen different genes are associated with Alzheimer's disease. Some are very common, and some are rare. Some nearly always cause Alzheimer's disease (top-left cluster of genes), whereas others are more common and increase risk modestly (*APOE*). Some are very common but change risk only slightly (bottom-right cluster).
(Figure adapted for use with permission and created by Alan Renton, PhD, and provided courtesy of Alison Goate, D.Phil, Icahn School of Medicine at Mount Sinai, New York, NY.)

neurologic examination. Bloodwork is done to look for reversible causes of dementia such as thyroid or vitamin deficiency. Brain imaging such as a CT scan or MRI of the brain looks for brain atrophy (shrinkage) and to rule out other issues such as a tumor or stroke. Traditionally, unless another cause was suggested in the diagnostic process, Alzheimer's disease is diagnosed at this point. As discussed in the last section and in Chapter 2, rarely genetic testing would be advised.

In 2021, the United States Food and Drug Administration (FDA) approved the first of what are hoped to be other new treatments for

Alzheimer's disease. In order for these drugs to work, these new treatments will likely require doctors to know if there is evidence of amyloid in the brain or not. This can be determined through an amyloid PET scan or a lumbar puncture, and possibly a blood test. Many neurologists have experience with ordering and understanding the results of these tests, and it is expected that knowing a person's amyloid status will become more important over time. However, these tests may only be ordered on those who are eligible for these treatments. Apolipoprotein E (APOE) is a gene that can impact the risk of developing Alzheimer's disease (see Chapter 2). But because APOE does not definitively cause Alzheimer's disease, prior to now people were not routinely tested for it. However, APOE strongly predicts responses to new amyloid treatment, so APOE testing may also become an important part of deciding if the new medications are safe and effective for someone to take (Chapter 10). PET scans, spinal fluid tests, and blood tests for tau are becoming available but are not part of deciding if someone can be treated with anti-amyloid treatments. The new treatments for Alzheimer's disease are discussed in more detail in Chapter 10.

Cognitive reserve and Alzheimer's disease

A fascinating unresolved issue in Alzheimer's disease is that some people demonstrate Alzheimer's symptoms while others do not, despite having the same amount of microscopic brain changes of the disease. One possible explanation is the concept of **cognitive reserve**. The theory is that people who have experienced more cognitively rich lifestyles across their lifespan are less likely to express symptoms of Alzheimer's disease even though they have Alzheimer's changes in the brain. Greater cognitive reserve is associated with a longer and richer educational history, professional attainment/job complexity, and cognitive enrichment throughout one's life. Cognitive reserve may result from strengthened **neural networks** that develop across the lifespan because of more cognitive stimulation and may enable the brain to compensate and function despite obvious brain changes. The theory of cognitive reserve suggests that early or midlife efforts to enhance cognitive reserve may reduce the risks of developing Alzheimer's disease. Not much is known about cognitive reserve in dementia aside from Alzheimer's disease, but most likely the same protective factors are important in other causes of dementia.

Because Alzheimer's disease is the most common form of dementia, other forms of dementia have been termed "non-Alzheimer's dementia." The next few chapters review how the non-Alzheimer's dementias (including dementia with Lewy bodies, frontotemporal dementia, and others) are identified and how these other disorders differ from Alzheimer's disease and from one another.

CHAPTER 6

Dementia with Lewy Bodies

In this chapter, you will learn about:

- Lewy body dementias, including dementia with Lewy bodies, and Parkinson's disease dementia
- The key clinical features and differences between dementia with Lewy bodies, Parkinson's disease dementia, and Alzheimer's disease
- What causes dementia with Lewy bodies
- How dementia with Lewy bodies is diagnosed

This chapter focuses on the second most common cause of dementia, dementia with Lewy bodies. Just as Alzheimer's disease is named for the changes first described by Dr. Alzheimer, the microscopic brain changes seen in Parkinson's disease that are now called "Lewy bodies" are named for Frederic Lewy, who first identified them in 1912. These changes are now known to be composed of clumped brain protein called α-synuclein. These clumps, which are known as **inclusion bodies**, appear microscopically in the nerve cells (Figure 6.1).

The changes seen in dementia with Lewy bodies are similar to the microscopic changes seen in Parkinson's disease but occur in different brain regions. Because very similar microscopic changes are seen in both diseases, some researchers consider Parkinson's disease and dementia with Lewy bodies to be on a continuum of a single disease occurring in different brain regions for reasons not currently understood. Lewy bodies are seen deep in the brain in Parkinson's disease,

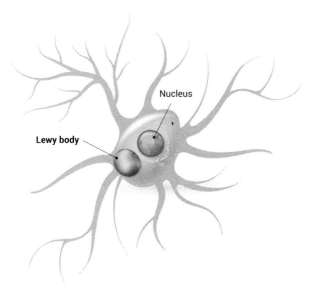

FIGURE 6.1 **Lewy body in a nerve cell.** Lewy bodies are round clumps of a protein called α-synuclein. Lewy bodies are seen in the nerve cells of the brains of people with Lewy body dementias and Parkinson's disease.

whereas they are seen in some regions of the cortex in dementia with Lewy bodies.

Several very similar and potentially confusing terms are worth defining. Lewy body dementia is a broad term that refers to a group of three dementias that have microscopic Lewy body changes in common and some overlapping features:

- Dementia with Lewy bodies (sometimes called diffuse Lewy body disease)
- Parkinson's disease dementia
- The Lewy body variant of Alzheimer's disease

Dementia with Lewy bodies is the second most common progressive dementia after Alzheimer's disease, but it is far less common than Alzheimer's disease. Dementia with Lewy bodies is estimated to occur in from 0.1% to 2% of persons older than 65 years of age, ranging from 1 in 1,000 to 1 in 50 people. This is just a small fraction of the figures for Alzheimer's disease, which affects close to 1 in 6 people older than 65 years of age. In contrast to Alzheimer's disease, dementia with Lewy bodies affects men more than women. About one-fourth of people with Alzheimer's disease also have microscopic Lewy body changes. People with both of these changes may have overlapping features and can have a faster progression and an earlier age of onset.

Signs and symptoms of dementia with Lewy bodies

Dementia with Lewy bodies presents as a mix of cognitive, behavioral, and, in particular, physical changes that help distinguish it from other forms of dementia such as Alzheimer's disease. Just as Alzheimer's disease can be different from one person to the next, dementia with Lewy bodies can present in different ways too. For example, in dementia with Lewy bodies, the physical changes sometimes do not begin until later in the disease; however, in many cases, the behavioral, cognitive, and motor symptoms begin around the same time.

Changes in mobility and balance in dementia with Lewy bodies

Parkinsonism describes a group of symptoms that includes stiffness, slowness, **tremor**, and problems with walking and balance (Figure 6.2). These parkinsonian symptoms are most often seen in Parkinson's disease but are also a hallmark of dementia with Lewy bodies, beginning within about a year of the onset of cognitive problems, although they can also develop years after cognitive and behavioral symptoms first begin. In contrast, obvious cognitive problems may be

Parkinson's Disease Symptoms

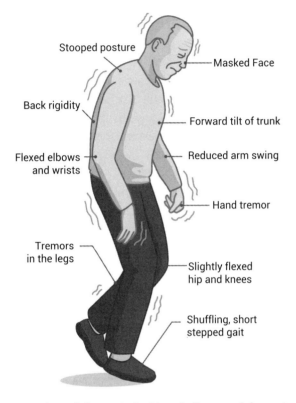

Stooped posture

Masked Face

Back rigidity

Forward tilt of trunk

Flexed elbows
and wrists

Reduced arm swing

Hand tremor

Tremors
in the legs

Slightly flexed
hip and knees

Shuffling, short
stepped gait

FIGURE 6.2 Physical changes in Parkinson's disease and dementia with Lewy bodies. Features of parkinsonism include tremor, stiffness, slowness, and gait instability. These are the primary features of Parkinson's disease and may present on one side of the body, particularly tremor, which is most noticeable at rest. In contrast, in dementia with Lewy bodies, parkinsonian features such as tremor tend to present on both sides at the same time, usually long after cognitive and behavioral changes begin.

seen in people with Parkinson's disease but usually not until years or even decades after the first symptoms. When dementia is diagnosed several years after Parkinson's disease is diagnosed, the condition is termed Parkinson's disease dementia. Parkinson's disease dementia can develop when Lewy bodies start to appear elsewhere in the brain or sometimes when a patient with Parkinson's disease also develops Alzheimer's disease. It is often difficult to determine the underlying changes in the brain when people have an advanced state of parkinsonism and cognitive changes.

Medications used in Parkinson's disease are usually not as effective for parkinsonism in dementia with Lewy bodies, and these medications may even worsen behavioral problems, especially hallucinations. However, behavioral symptoms may be controlled with antipsychotic medications (Chapter 11). Parkinsonism typically progresses along with cognitive problems in the course of dementia with Lewy bodies. Compared to Alzheimer's disease, physical support needs often occur earlier and become more apparent with time in both dementia with Lewy bodies and Parkinson's disease dementia.

Cognitive impairment

Dementia with Lewy bodies often shares the cognitive features of Alzheimer's disease but with some important differences. Similar to Alzheimer's disease, memory often seems to be affected in dementia with Lewy bodies. But neuropsychological testing (Chapter 2) shows that patients with dementia with Lewy bodies tend to have more executive or visuospatial problems than those with Alzheimer's disease. These visuospatial problems are not the same as the prominent visual hallucinations seen in dementia with Lewy bodies (discussed further in the next section). Cognitive abilities and motor symptoms can vary dramatically from one day to the next; affected persons may seem strikingly clear or lucid on some days compared to others. These swings in cognitive and motor abilities are called **fluctuations**. Sometimes when fluctuations are dramatic, patients may be misdiagnosed with seizures, especially when hallucinations are present, but an **electroencephalogram** (a brainwave test for seizures also known as **EEG**) does not find any seizures.

Behavioral and psychological symptoms

Dementia with Lewy bodies has two other distinctive features: hallucinations and dramatic changes in sleep. Visual hallucinations are common in dementia with Lewy bodies and take on the form of seeing people, animals, or insects in a room. Sometimes people with dementia with Lewy bodies may misperceive something seen in the room; for instance, they may misinterpret a couch pillow as a cat or a pattern on the floor as a crawling insect. This is called an **illusion**. Other times, people with dementia with Lewy bodies may think they see something just out of the corner of their eye; this is called a **sensed presence**. Visual symptoms may become more complex and may have some features of Alzheimer's disease, including delusions; for instance, patients may perceive that someone on the television news or on a virtual meeting is with them in the room. Sometimes more complex visual hallucinations can occur, such as seeing a family member who has passed away. In contrast to Alzheimer's disease, personality changes are rare, although depression and apathy may occur.

Another unique feature of dementia of Lewy bodies is very active (and sometimes disruptive) sleep, which is noticed by others as more than just tossing and turning. These changes are collectively known as **rapid eye movement (REM) sleep behavior disorder** and can be particularly disruptive in dementia with Lewy bodies, causing phenomena such as sleeptalking (also known as **somniloquy**) and acting out dreams (**dream enactment**). Sometimes bed partners will be struck during a violent dream, and sometimes the person with dementia with Lewy bodies may fall out of bed or break furniture and injure themselves. The reasons for these changes are complex. Ordinarily in the earliest stages of sleep, the brain is in a transitional stage between fully awake and the deeper restorative periods of sleep. A normal part of sleep known as **rapid eye movement (REM)** sleep is unique in that during this stage, the brain is very active and the eyes rapidly jerk in all directions while the body is still. It is thought that an area of the brainstem responsible for stopping all limb and bodily movements during REM sleep becomes uncoupled from its normal circuit in persons with dementia with Lewy bodies. When this happens, REM sleep behavior disorder develops.

REM sleep behaviors such as these also occur in healthy people and may be side effects of certain medications, including some antidepressant medications. Other types of sleep problems are common throughout life. Brief limb jerks are common and usually normal. Many children have physically active sleep that may include sleepwalking (also known as **somnambulism**), sleeptalking, and nightmares, and these should not cause alarm or concern for dementia. In dementia with Lewy bodies, REM sleep changes may predate other cognitive or physical symptoms by years. During the daytime, visual hallucinations can have an appearance of sleep, and periods of dream-like visual hallucinations can occur. The medical treatment of REM sleep behavior disorder is discussed in Chapter 11, and nighttime safety is discussed in Chapter 14.

David is 68 and began having vivid dreams and talking in his sleep about 10 years ago, first noticed by his wife of 42 years. Two years ago, he began having episodes of thinking that he was seeing children but just out of the corner of his eye; they always disappeared when he tried to find them. Ten months ago, David and his wife noticed that he had been falling often, his walking speed had slowed, and his handwriting had become small and difficult to read. He was referred for physical therapy, which helped only modestly. An orthopedist found no evidence that arthritis was causing his imbalance. About 3 months ago, his family began to notice a big difference in his mental clarity from one day to another, without any explanation. Last week, he began seeing birds flying in his apartment; his family brings this to the attention of his primary care physician.

(Continued)

(Continued)

The medical examination reveals that David has memory loss and difficulty with copying even simple drawings. His posture is stooped when he walks, and he nearly falls when turning too quickly and when attempting to sit in a chair. Laboratory tests and imaging are unremarkable, including showing no brain atrophy on the MRI. Based on the closely timed onset of parkinsonism and dementia with complex visual hallucinations as well as REM sleep behavior disorder, David is diagnosed with dementia with Lewy bodies.

Other signs and symptoms in dementia with Lewy bodies

The autonomic nervous system (Chapter 4) is often involved in dementia with Lewy bodies and sometimes early in the course of disease. Persons with either dementia with Lewy bodies or Parkinson's disease dementia may experience serious problems with fainting spells and constipation. Urinary control issues may occur earlier in the course of disease than in Alzheimer's disease. As is the case with other symptoms of dementia, it can be hard to distinguish some problems of the autonomic nervous system from normal changes of aging or even from possible side effects from medications taken for non-neurologic reasons.

Parkinson's disease dementia: a close relative of dementia with Lewy bodies

Sonja is a 78-year-old woman who has had a very successful career in graphic design. She retired 15 years ago because of the onset of a Parkinson's disease tremor that impacted her drafting

(Continued)

(Continued)

skills and dexterity. Nonetheless, in retirement she has enjoyed painting and spending time with her husband. About 2 years ago, her husband began to notice that she had some trouble composing her paintings and had difficulty interpreting how some objects related to one another when trying to paint a still life; at about the same time, she started to have trouble remembering recent conversations. Her husband recently has started helping her remember when it's time to take medications. She got lost while driving to the grocery store 2 weeks ago although they have lived in the same town for years. At their next neurologist visit, they discuss these new concerns, and a diagnostic evaluation for dementia is pursued, including brain imaging. She is diagnosed with Parkinson's disease dementia.

Parkinson's disease dementia and dementia with Lewy bodies are thought to exist on a continuum, and sometimes making a clinical distinction between the two can be difficult. However, distinguishing between the two has implications for treatment, including how the motor symptoms may be treated in one compared to the other. For more about Parkinson's disease, refer to the book *Navigating Life with Parkinson's Disease, Second Edition* by Sotirios Parashos, MD, PHD, and Rose Wichman, PT (Oxford University Press, 2020), in this series.

What causes dementia with Lewy bodies?

What causes dementia with Lewy bodies remains uncertain. Because it is much less common than Alzheimer's disease, the amount that is known about dementia with Lewy bodies lags far behind what is known about Alzheimer's disease, including its causes, risk factors, specific diagnostic testing, and genetics. Although the brain changes of Parkinson's disease are better understood, its causes also remain uncertain, except in persons with rare genetic causes. The microscopic changes of Parkinson's disease and dementia with Lewy bodies are similar, but the reasons for these changes appear to be quite different and may be unrelated.

Diagnostic testing for dementia with Lewy bodies

The time from initial evaluation to correct diagnosis in patients with dementia with Lewy bodies is often longer than in Alzheimer's disease. This likely relates to the overlapping features of dementia with Lewy bodies, Alzheimer's disease, and Parkinson's disease and to less general awareness of dementia with Lewy bodies. Further, about one-third of people with Alzheimer's disease will develop some features of dementia with Lewy bodies and have microscopic Lewy body changes. When this occurs, the disease is called the **Lewy body variant of Alzheimer's disease**.

When doctors suspect dementia with Lewy bodies, they will typically request a workup similar to that of Alzheimer's disease and other dementias, including taking a history, performing physical and neurologic examinations, and ordering laboratory work and brain imaging such as a CT or MRI and sometimes a dopamine transporter scan (Chapter 2). Given newly available treatments for Alzheimer's disease, the diagnostic workup may also include testing for amyloid in the brain through PET, spinal fluid, and possibly bloodwork (see Chapters 2 and 5). As in Alzheimer's disease, not much may be found on testing despite a comprehensive search. Specific to dementia with Lewy bodies, although profound symptoms may be present at the time of an evaluation, an MRI may appear relatively normal with only minimal atrophy. A dopamine transporter scan will be positive in dementia with Lewy bodies and Parkinson's disease dementia but negative in Alzheimer's disease.

CHAPTER 7

Frontotemporal Dementia

In this chapter, you will learn about:

- The spectrum of the frontotemporal dementias
- How to identify the key signs and symptoms of common forms of frontotemporal dementia, including language and behavioral changes, and how they differ from other forms of dementia
- How frontotemporal dementias are diagnosed

As previously discussed, dementia is an umbrella term capturing many different causes. Frontotemporal dementia (FTD), also referred to as frontotemporal lobar degeneration, is also an umbrella term used to capture several less common forms of dementia with overlapping symptoms, microscopic changes, and genetic causes. Two main forms of FTD exist: a behavioral form (behavioral variant FTD) and a language form (primary progressive aphasia). Either form may be accompanied by parkinsonism or a disorder of muscle weakness called amyotrophic lateral sclerosis (ALS) (also known as Lou Gehrig's disease or motor neuron disease). Less common are forms of FTD that can present primarily with physical decline, including corticobasal syndrome and progressive supranuclear palsy (PSP).

FTD is a group of diseases that have some overlapping clinical features but are not described by a single microscopic brain change. Instead, multiple types and combinations of clumped brain proteins known as tau and TDP-43 are seen. In recent years, there has been a push to define FTD disorders based on not only the microscopic brain changes but also the types of proteins and genes. However, from a practical perspective, it is helpful to think about how doctors view the various symptoms of FTD. Figure 7.1 breaks down the different forms of the FTD spectrum and how the disorders are named based on signs, symptoms, and findings on neuropsychological assessments, lab testing, and imaging.

Overall, FTD is the fourth most common dementia, causing less than 5% of all dementia cases, but it is the third most common neurodegenerative dementia after Alzheimer's disease and dementia with Lewy bodies. Onset tends to be younger than other dementias, and before age 65, FTD is as common as Alzheimer's disease. Although estimates are sparse, approximately 2 per 100,000 to 15 per 100,000 people aged 65 years and younger are thought to have FTD. Like other forms of dementia, the earliest symptoms often determine how the doctor makes the diagnosis of an FTD. In some forms of FTD, behavioral or personality changes are seen before or at the same time as cognitive changes. Poor speech fluency is another clue. Neuropsychological testing (Chapter 2) can be especially helpful in identifying executive or language dysfunction in FTD. Memory loss

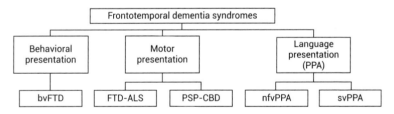

FIGURE 7.1 Organization of FTD based on clinical presentation. FTD may present with changes in 1 of 3 primary areas: behavioral, motor, or language. Within each of these areas are sub-forms of frontotemporal dementia, often with overlapping features. Abbreviations: bvFTD (behavioral variant FTD), CBD (corticobasal degeneration), FTD-ALS (FTD with ALS), nfvPPA (nonfluent variant primary progressive aphasia, also known as progressive nonfluent aphasia), PPA (primary progressive aphasia), PSP (progressive supranuclear palsy), svPPA (semantic variant primary progressive aphasia, also known as semantic dementia).

is common in FTD, but most people with FTD have relative sparing of visuospatial function. MRI of patients with FTD reveals atrophy in frontal and temporal lobes, in contrast to patients with Alzheimer's disease, who more often have changes in the size and shape of parietal and temporal lobes (Chapter 4). FDG-PET, a form of functional neuroimaging, can help identify the brain regions that are affected in FTD (Chapter 2).

Behavioral and language presentations of FTD

The two most common forms of FTD are disorders of behavior and executive function (behavioral variant FTD) and, less often, a disorder of language called primary progressive aphasia (including progressive nonfluent aphasia and semantic dementia). In the past, behavioral variant FTD was called Pick's disease, named for the physician who discovered the disease in 1892, but this term has fallen out of favor and has been replaced by more specific terms describing the clinical syndrome. However, the term Pick's disease or Pick's bodies may still be used when describing certain underlying microscopic changes.

Hallmarks of behavioral variant FTD include dysfunction of the frontal lobes of the brain, including changes in attention and concentration, problems organizing thoughts, and profound personality changes. Memory may be affected, but memory changes are typically less apparent in earlier stages. Behavioral features may include obsessive-compulsive features with odd rituals or habits, changes in relating to other people, lack of empathy, irritability, and uncontrollable sadness or laughter. The behavioral symptoms in FTD may be subtle at onset but often come to define the illness. Often people with Alzheimer's disease are poorly aware of their symptoms but may be upset when discussing them with others. In contrast, those with FTD may not care even when confronted with a diagnosis. The behavioral changes, especially changes in social awareness and personality, may be exhausting for the family and caregivers, and many symptoms can be difficult (but not impossible) to control with medications and complementary supportive approaches.

> *Elizabeth is a 45-year-old woman whose husband notes that she has developed some peculiar behaviors in recent months, including very specific food preferences. Her day is not complete unless she has a specific brand of cake every day at lunch. She has always been very friendly, but now she kisses everyone she meets, making others uncomfortable. Along with her obsessions and personality changes, she has trouble focusing and speaks more slowly than in the past. Although Elizabeth isn't bothered by her symptoms, her husband is and arranges for her to see a specialist. A similar illness affected her father, who died of a non-Alzheimer's dementia in his early 60s, and her older sister has recently become estranged because she has developed problems with alcohol use later in life. A detailed neurologic examination reveals that Elizabeth is having difficulty understanding simple proverbs and shifting from one thought to another, and she is unable to perform simple arithmetic. Her attempts to embrace and kiss the physician disrupt the office visit repeatedly. MRI reveals substantial atrophy in both frontal regions of the brain, and a diagnosis of behavioral FTD is made.*

When language problems are the principal symptoms of FTD, it is called primary progressive aphasia. Similar symptoms may be seen abruptly after a stroke, but in FTD, aphasia develops gradually, usually over months to years. Aphasia in FTD most often presents as a nonfluent aphasia, and as the name suggests there is a loss of fluency, or the ease with which someone speaks. Instead, gradual but noticeable changes emerge, with disrupted, halting, or disjointed speech becoming apparent. Someone with nonfluent aphasia may appear frustrated when they speak, and others may try to complete their sentences or fill in the blanks to help communicate thoughts. In nonfluent aphasia, written and heard speech can still be understood by the person with aphasia. Another less common form of aphasia in FTD that also develops gradually is called semantic dementia. Semantic dementia involves difficulty understanding the semantics, or meaning, of words. Sometimes persons with semantic dementia can readily identify objects but cannot describe their characteristics or details. For example, someone with semantic dementia may have difficulty describing the purpose of a shopping cart or whether or not they like Swiss cheese, although they can easily name them. Like the different presentations of dementia, aphasia in FTD can have many variations. Elizabeth's story is typical of someone with behavioral variant FTD. FTD can have overlapping features of both behavioral and language forms.

> *Frieda is a 54-year-old executive who began having trouble expressing herself in work meetings about a year ago, and the difficulty has worsened in recent months. Her family notices that she is withdrawn at family gatherings and sometimes struggles to speak when everyone is together. Her father died of a non-Alzheimer's dementia in his 60s, about 30 years ago. Her physician begins a workup and refers her to a neurologist. Her MRI reveals frontal and temporal atrophy, and neuropsychological testing supports a diagnosis of progressive nonfluent aphasia and FTD. Her family is interested in genetic testing and discusses it with her doctor.*

PSP and corticobasal degeneration

Although persons with FTD may later develop the physical changes of parkinsonism, two additional diseases fall into the FTD spectrum (see Figure 7.1) and primarily present with the physical changes of parkinsonism, such as slowing, stiffness, tremor, and problems with walking and balance (Chapter 6). The first, PSP, is associated with changes in vertical eye movements and balance, particularly with significant problems with falling backward. Other features include changes in facial expression and swallowing. It is now recognized that the brain changes of PSP are associated with a broader range of symptoms, including FTD behavioral changes, before the physical changes of parkinsonism begin. Many people with typical PSP develop features of an FTD-like dementia as the disease progresses. One particular clinical feature seen in PSP is called pseudobulbar affect, with the hallmark of uncontrollable laughter or crying.

Eugene is a 61-year-old man who has worked as a janitor in a local school for 30 years. Over the past year, he developed problems with balance, initially attributed to arthritis in his knees. Last week, he fell backward at work and was not able to protect himself, striking his head as he fell. After a brief hospitalization, he is evaluated by a neurologist, who notes additional history. Over the past year, Eugene's voice has become quieter, his walking has slowed, and he has developed difficulty concentrating. His neurologic examination shows that he has trouble looking vertically up and down, and all his eye movements are slower. MRI shows that his midbrain region is much smaller than expected. Over the next 6 months, his symptoms worsen, especially his balance. He is eventually diagnosed with PSP and has to retire. Medications used for Parkinson's disease are tried but only partially relieve the stiffness. Physical therapy has been helpful with learning how to avoid falls and use a walker but has not helped his balance. Eugene's sister steps in to help manage his affairs, and a home health aide is hired to reduce his risk of falls.

Corticobasal degeneration, sometimes referred to as the FTD form of corticobasal syndrome, is a rare form of FTD that typically presents with a complex set of symptoms suggesting one-sided or asymmetric changes in motor function. The placement by scientists of corticobasal degeneration in the FTD spectrum rather than the Alzheimer's spectrum continues to evolve. Clinical features can be very similar to the corticobasal syndrome form of Alzheimer's disease but with much more profound asymmetry in arm or hand function in FTD. These changes, when profound, are called an "alien" limb since control of movement becomes increasingly difficult and movements may occur spontaneously with no voluntary component. Corticobasal degeneration may be associated with profound parkinsonism; otherwise, the clinical features have substantial overlap with other forms of dementia, particularly in later stages.

Motor neuron disease in FTD

In most forms of dementia, the spinal cord and the peripheral nerves are not part of the dementia process. But in some people, the nerve cells in the spinal cord that help move the muscles (the motor neurons) can become diseased in a process similar to the one affecting brain cells, leading to weakness due to ALS. ALS is likely the third most common neurodegenerative disease behind Alzheimer's disease and Parkinson's disease. ALS is thought to develop in about 10% to 15% of persons with FTD, especially in persons with one of the genetic or inherited forms of FTD. Symptoms of ALS include severe progressive muscle weakness that may begin in one part of the body, such as one hand or one leg, eventually spreading to involve nearly all muscles under voluntary control, including those used for swallowing and breathing. Many people with ALS may also have mild cognitive and behavioral features as seen in FTD. But because ALS tends to progress rapidly, the FTD symptoms may be relatively minor and overlooked, especially in the early stages. Later, when the physical problems of

ALS limit mobility and social engagement, behavioral and cognitive problems continue to be difficult to detect.

> *Helena is a 58-year-old executive who notices that her right leg is somewhat clumsy one day while on a jog. Later that month, she has trouble going up the stairs, especially with her right foot. After speaking with her primary care physician, an MRI of her brain and spinal cord is performed. Since the imaging is normal, she is referred to a neurologist. She is seen several months into her illness, by which time her left arm is also clumsy and her hand grip is weak. Findings on the examination raise concern for ALS, which is later supported by testing of her nerves and muscles with electromyography and nerve conduction studies. Her father died at age 63 of a non-Alzheimer's dementia. Genetic testing is positive and explains Helena's ALS with cognitive problems as well as her father's presumed FTD. As part of her care, Helena enters a research trial for people with genetic causes of ALS.*

Further information about ALS is available in another book in this series, *Navigating Life with Amyotrophic Lateral Sclerosis* by Mark B. Bromberg, MD, PhD, FAAN, and Diane Banks Bromberg, JD (Oxford University Press, 2017).

Diagnostic testing for FTD

The diagnostic process for FTD shares some features with people being evaluated for Alzheimer's disease and dementia with Lewy bodies. Doctors will typically begin by taking a history, performing physical and neurologic examinations, and ordering laboratory work and brain imaging such as a CT or MRI. FTD may show distinctive changes on brain imaging, but often there are overlapping features with Alzheimer's disease. Because some clinical and imaging features in FTD may be confused with Alzheimer's disease, additional diagnostic testing is often done. Testing can include FDG-PET, which is helpful in distinguishing Alzheimer's disease from FTD. Additional testing can include spinal fluid analysis for amyloid and tau biomarkers (Chapter 2). Since there is no spinal fluid biomarker profile specific to FTD but there is for Alzheimer's disease, a lumbar puncture is done primarily to make sure that biomarkers do not instead suggest an unusual presentation of Alzheimer's disease. In people with FTD who also have suspected ALS, an electromyogram may be ordered. Genetic testing is much more commonly pursued in FTD.

Genetic testing in FTD

FTD is unique in that about one-third of all people with FTD will have a family history suspicious for genetic causes of dementia. Several genes have been implicated in FTD, the most common being *C9orf72*, *MAPT*, and *GRN*. Several others are known to exist but are much

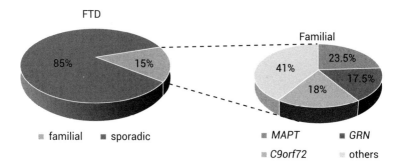

FIGURE 7.2 **Genetic causes of FTD.** About 10% to 15% of cases of FTD have a known genetic basis. The three most common genes, *MAPT*, *GRN*, and *C9orf72*, make up about 60% of these. Because FTD often has a genetic basis, genetic testing is often discussed in the course of evaluation and treatment. *Source*: Frontiers In Bioscience, Landmark, 23, 1144-1165, January 1, 2018.

rarer, and the list continues to grow. For about 10% of persons with FTD, an identifiable genetic cause for FTD will be found through conventional genetic testing even if no family history is known. Because these genes are so frequently found in FTD, genetic testing is more often discussed and considered in FTD than in other dementias. The role of genetic counseling in advance of genetic testing is discussed in Chapter 2. Figure 7.2 highlights the complex relationships between the clinical features of FTD and their genetics.

CHAPTER 8

Vascular Dementia

In this chapter, you will learn about:

- The key clinical features of vascular dementia
- The differences between the different types of vascular dementia: single-infarct dementia, subcortical white matter disease, and cerebral amyloid angiopathy
- The importance of controlling vascular risk factors in preventing stroke

Stroke is a common neurologic problem, affecting about 3% of people at some point in their lifetime. Strokes happen when a blood vessel in the brain is blocked or broken. Strokes cause sudden changes in physical function or sensation of a limb or side of the body, may cause changes in vision, and sometimes can cause memory and other cognitive problems, depending on where the stroke occurs. Stroke is comprehensively covered in another volume in this series, *Navigating the Complexities of Stroke* by Louis R. Caplan, MD, FAAN (Oxford University Press, 2013); this chapter discusses how stroke can lead to cognitive impairment and dementia.

From examination of the brain on autopsy, it is recognized that about one in three older people die with at least one stroke, but most never show symptoms. Most strokes occur due to a blockage of blood vessels (ischemic stroke). Less often, a stroke results from a rupture of a blood vessel in the brain (**hemorrhagic stroke**). When one stroke or multiple strokes affect brain regions that are important for cognition or behavior, vascular dementia results. Figure 8.1 shows what happens in the brain in ischemic and hemorrhagic stroke.

Vascular dementia is the third most common cause of dementia (after Alzheimer's disease and dementia with Lewy bodies). Dementia can result from strokes in three different ways: **large single cerebral**

Brain Stroke

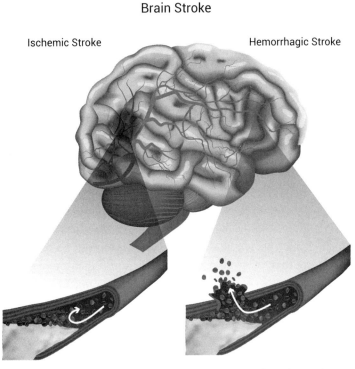

FIGURE 8.1 **Primary types of stroke.** Stroke generally occurs with a disruption of blood in the brain because of either a rupture or blockage of a blood vessel. These changes can occur in large or small blood vessels. Vascular dementia develops when one or more large strokes occur in areas important for cognition or after multiple small strokes together cause similar changes.

Cerebrovascular disease	Changes in the brain	Dementia types
Atherosclerosis	Large territory strokes, ischemic or hemorrhagic	Single infarct dementia Multi-infarct dementia
Small vessel ischemic disease	Small territory strokes, in white matter or deep in the brain	Multi-infarct dementia Subcortical white matter disease
Cerebral amyloid angiopathy	Hemorrhagic strokes in cerebrum, small and large territory	Multi-infarct dementia Single infarct dementia

FIGURE 8.2 Vascular dementia and its causes. Three general categories of stroke can lead to dementia: large single cerebral infarctions (either ischemic or hemorrhagic strokes), multiple small vessel strokes in the white matter, and multiple small hemorrhages (known as cerebral amyloid angiopathy), which are often seen in Alzheimer's disease.

infarctions, subcortical white matter microvascular disease, and cerebral amyloid angiopathy (CAA). Each has a distinct pattern of presenting signs and symptoms. Figure 8.2 shows the relationship between the three main causes of cerebrovascular disease, the types of microscopic changes seen, and the clinically defined forms of vascular dementia.

Altogether, vascular dementia is responsible for a small proportion of dementia in Europe and the United States, but may be responsible for as much as 15% of dementia in Asian populations. The reason for this discrepancy is unclear. Vascular dementia is much more likely to occur in people who have vascular risk factors such as coronary heart disease or its causes, including diabetes, hypertension, elevated cholesterol, or smoking tobacco. **Atrial fibrillation**, a disorder of the heart's rhythm, is also a major risk factor for stroke and vascular dementia.

Large single-infarct dementia

The most obvious stroke-associated dementia is one that follows a large or catastrophic stroke. Large single-infarct dementia refers to a single major stroke that may leave someone suddenly disabled and dependent upon others. Because of this new dependence on others (Chapter 1), this new poststroke state is also considered dementia. This type of dementia is especially common after someone has a stroke in brain regions principally responsible for how language is made or understood. Strokes of similar size in other areas of the brain may cause major physically disabling changes but do not affect cognition or behavior and thus are not called dementia. However, because some large strokes affect language or memory or lead to other cognitive problems, dementia can be seen after a stroke. Sometimes people can have several large strokes in their lifetime that together cause accumulated injury to the brain and thus cause vascular dementia.

Darryl is a 62-year-old man with uncontrolled diabetes, hypertension, and a heart arrhythmia called atrial fibrillation. He often doesn't take the medications prescribed for these conditions. While home alone one day, he develops the inability to speak or move his right arm or feel the side of his face. An hour later, his grandson arrives home from school and quickly recognizes that his grandfather may be having a stroke based on face and arm weakness and his inability to speak. His grandson dials 911, and within 2 hours of stroke onset, Darryl is examined at the local hospital and receives tissue plasminogen activator, known as the "clot buster" medication. Three months after the stroke, he has had only modest recovery in language, whereas his right arm has gotten much stronger over time. Because of his aphasia following the stroke, Darryl cannot express himself well and has some trouble understanding others. He needs help with shopping, errands, and managing his finances and is diagnosed with vascular dementia.

Subcortical strokes and dementia

Deep within the brain in the **subcortical** areas lie the **white matter** regions of the brain, which serve as information pathways connecting one part of the brain to another. If one of these paths is cut, as can happen in a small **ischemic** or **hemorrhagic stroke**, it may not be obvious. But after many small subcortical strokes, these changes accumulate to cause **subcortical white matter disease** or multiple small cerebral infarctions deep in the brain. Unless a stroke occurs deep in the brain in a targeted spot that causes weakness in the arm, face, or leg, these deep subcortical strokes may be "silent," or difficult to be noticed by the patient or the doctor. However, the net effect of many subcortical strokes is slow mental processing speed, problems with paying attention and staying focused, and depressive symptoms. Although subtle, sometimes a stepwise pattern of changes (see Figure 3.1) is noted in retrospect rather than a slow steady process as is seen in Alzheimer's disease. When strokes and Alzheimer's disease are both present, memory problems are likely to begin at an earlier age and the cumulative problem is worse than with either condition alone.

Richard is a 58-year-old man with poorly controlled hypertension. He has had two strokes in the past 3 years, resulting in clumsiness of his left hand and foot. His sister has noticed that over the past few years he has become depressed and takes a lot longer to understand when something is explained to him. Twice in the past year, these changes have suddenly worsened from one week to the next. He had to give up his electrician job a few weeks ago because he was unable to troubleshoot simple problems. Once he forgot to deactivate a circuit, and his partner suffered an electrical injury. In the past, workup for his strokes identified numerous small subcortical strokes. His primary care physician suspects that he has vascular dementia due to subcortical white matter disease and that he is forgetting to take his blood pressure medication. His sister begins to help out in managing his care.

Cerebral amyloid angiopathy

CAA is a third form of vascular dementia. CAA causes hemorrhagic strokes, both small and large, that are sometimes only seen on MRI. It is distinguished from other types of hemorrhagic strokes since CAA is caused by brain changes similar to those caused by amyloid in Alzheimer's disease (Chapter 5). Amyloid may also aggregate and accumulate in the walls of brain blood vessels. Nearly every time that Alzheimer's disease is diagnosed, these vascular amyloid changes are also seen. However, amyloid deposition in the vessel walls may not cause obvious symptoms until a significant brain **hemorrhage** (bleeding stroke) occurs. After a brain hemorrhage occurs, MRI may show previous brain bleeds that were not obvious by prior history alone. As with single-infarct dementia, these hemorrhagic strokes cause specific types of symptoms principally based upon their brain location. Some of the newer medications that treat the amyloid-related biological changes of Alzheimer's disease have been associated with inflammation and small hemorrhagic strokes similar to what is seen in CAA, and this is covered further in Chapter 10.

Sarah is a 72-year-old woman who began having mild memory loss over the past year. Her doctor believes she may have a form of Alzheimer's disease. One morning while they're having breakfast, her husband notices that she has trouble talking to him and understanding him. She holds her head in her hands as if she has a bad headache. He calls 911, and after she arrives at the hospital, a head CT shows she has a large left-sided brain bleed in an area important for language. Her blood pressure has never been a problem and remains normal throughout her hospitalization. An MRI is performed during her hospitalization, revealing more than a dozen small previous brain bleeds, and she is diagnosed with cerebral amyloid angiopathy.

Genetic forms of vascular dementia

Although rare, some genes may increase the risk of stroke in young people, and others can cause many strokes or strokes in unusual places in the brain. Several genes may increase the risk of developing clots in the veins, and these genes may be investigated following a stroke in a young person without conventional risk factors such as diabetes, hypertension, or heart disease. One example of genetic causes of vascular dementia is called **CADASIL** (**cerebral autosomal dominant arteriopathy with subcortical infarcts and leukoencephalopathy**). The frequency of CADASIL in the adult population is uncertain, but it is thought to occur in about 2 to 4 per 100,000 people. In families affected by CADASIL, it presents as an **autosomal dominant** inherited dementia, with half of each generation affected by the disease. Aside from a gradually progressive dementia, key features include subcortical strokes in unusual places, sometimes beginning in early to middle adulthood, that are accompanied by frequent headaches.

Preventing vascular dementia and delaying its progression

Vascular cognitive impairment related to a single large stroke or multiple subcortical strokes is unique since it's one of the main treatable and preventable forms of dementia. It is also one of the few forms of dementia in which the course is relatively static, unless, of course, more strokes happen. The risk factors for stroke are shown in Figure 8.3; the most common risk factors are high blood pressure, diabetes, high cholesterol, and inactivity. If the risk factors that result in stroke are controlled and new strokes are prevented, further cognitive decline can be prevented or delayed. Sometimes people with vascular dementia eventually develop progressive cognitive changes suggestive of Alzheimer's disease. In this situation, cognitive decline may result from a combination of stroke and Alzheimer's disease.

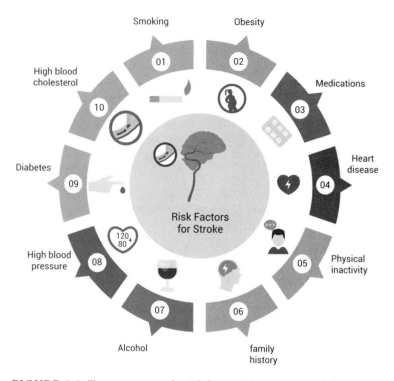

FIGURE 8.3 Ten common stroke risk factors. Many of these risk factors are often discussed and managed by a primary care physician. Addressing any one of these risk factors can decrease the chances of getting a stroke and therefore decrease stroke-related cognitive impairment. Even people with a prior history of stroke can cut down their risk for future stroke by controlling stroke risk factors.

Sometimes subtle stroke-like changes in the white matter are seen on brain scans even when the patient has had no symptoms of stroke. These changes are especially seen in people with a strong history of vascular risk factors, such as diabetes, hypertension, and smoking, but may also be seen in the brains of people without any risk factors. In addition to treating stroke risk factors, stroke itself is now treatable when recognized quickly after symptom onset (within a few hours, and every minute counts). Acute treatment options include intravenous medications (tissue plasminogen activator, or TPA) to break down clots or **thrombectomy** (mechanical removal of a brain clot by a special procedure). When vascular risk factors are recognized early, stroke may be preventable, dramatically reducing the risk of developing vascular dementia. To reduce the risk of stroke in the long term, some people may be prescribed certain blood thinners such as aspirin, or an anticoagulant medication.

So far, the focus of this book has been on the most common forms of dementia from neurodegenerative to vascular causes. The next chapter discusses rare causes of dementia, including rapidly progressive dementia.

CHAPTER 9

Less Common Causes of Dementia

In this chapter, you will learn about:

- Less common forms of neurodegenerative dementia
- The cognitive complications of other neurologic disorders, including multiple sclerosis and epilepsy
- The links between depression, schizophrenia, and dementia
- Potentially treatable or reversible forms of dementia
- Rapidly progressive dementias, including inflammatory brain diseases
- How the many forms of dementia compare and contrast with one another

Although Alzheimer's disease, dementia with Lewy bodies, frontotemporal dementia, and vascular dementia are most common, other dementias that are less common may be discussed with you and your family when you see a neurologist for evaluation of cognitive changes. These less common forms of dementia can be broadly grouped as rare genetic causes (**Huntington's disease**), **structural causes of dementia** (brain tumor, **subdural hematomas**, and **normal pressure hydrocephalus**), dementia due to other chronic neurologic disorders (including **multiple sclerosis**, **epilepsy**, and **schizophrenia**), autoimmune or acute inflammatory brain diseases, and rapidly progressive neurodegenerative diseases (including Creutzfeldt–Jakob disease [CJD]). Rarely, brain infections can also cause dementia. Sometimes causes of reversible cognitive impairment may be identified in the course of a dementia workup.

Some causes include compromised kidney or liver function, **vitamin B₁₂ deficiency**, **thyroid disease**, and depression, and this is covered in Chapter 2.

Huntington's disease

Huntington's disease is an uncommon exclusively genetic cause of dementia, occurring in approximately 7 per 100,000 people, with a presumed highest prevalence among those of European ancestry. Unlike many other disorders, the gene causing Huntington's disease is prone to replication and expansion when passed from one generation to the next. The increasing genetic expansion is associated with increasing disease severity and an earlier onset. As in other autosomal dominant diseases, half of the children of an affected person are at risk for developing the disease. Because of the genetic repeat expansion from one generation to the next, the age of onset can vary widely; onset may occur at a younger age than in the parent when the gene is from the father but at a similar age when passed from the mother. For this reason, Huntington's disease may occur in families without a strong family history, especially if passed through a father who may have died at a relatively young age. The symptoms are a unique combination of changes in movement and coordination, psychosis, and cognitive impairment, with problems with executive function early on and dementia later in the course. Through highly coordinated research efforts and strong engagement from many affected families, new approaches to treatment are being explored with encouraging preliminary results. Genetic counseling (Chapter 2) is an important part of care and planning in Huntington's disease.

Creutzfeldt–Jakob disease

CJD comprises three related disorders: a sporadic form, a genetic form, and variant or transmissible form. CJD typically presents as a rapidly progressive dementia that develops over weeks to months. A dramatic acceleration in the disease course may be seen, especially in later stages, when decline is noticeable day by day. Sporadic CJD is a rare form of dementia occurring in approximately 1 per 1,000,000 Americans and in about 6 per 1,000,000 over the age of 65. Sporadic CJD is clinically distinct from "variant" CJD, which affects younger persons and is primarily transmitted through donated human tissue unknowingly affected by CJD. Previously, variant CJD was associated with consumption of beef from cattle affected by "mad cow disease" or **bovine spongiform encephalopathy.** No cases of mad cow-associated variant CJD began in the United States, and new international cases are now rare if not altogether gone since livestock monitoring programs were introduced. Some symptoms of sporadic CJD can appear similar to other dementias, including problems with cognition, gait, visuospatial function, or balance. Sometimes severe pain or unusual sensory symptoms may occur. CJD is distinct from all other neurodegenerative dementias by its very rapidly progressive course, which can last only weeks to months and rarely more than a year from first symptom to death. CJD is diagnosed by specific MRI, cerebrospinal fluid, and electroencephalography (EEG) findings, without evidence of infection or inflammation in the cerebrospinal fluid. Sometimes CJD diagnostic testing will include a brain biopsy in hopes of finding something treatable. CJD has a number of different names based on the main presenting symptoms, including balance and coordination (**Gerstmann–Sträussler–Scheinker syndrome**), profound visuospatial symptoms (**Heidenhain variant**), or severe insomnia (**fatal familial insomnia**). Although rare, genetic forms of CJD with autosomal dominant patterns of inheritance exist, and some families may show different types of CJD syndromes among affected individuals. Unfortunately, there are no known treatments for any form of CJD.

Structural causes of dementia

Structural causes of dementia are a group of diseases in which large masses in the brain or excessive fluid retained in the brain compress or invade the brain and cause cognitive impairment. Some of these structural brain changes can be treated surgically, potentially stopping or slowing the cognitive changes seen.

Brain tumor–associated dementia

Dementia can be caused by a brain tumor when the mass disrupts brain regions that are involved in cognitive function. Brain tumors may occur in the brain as metastases from cancers that travel through the blood to the brain after starting in another part of the body (e.g., lung, breast, or colon), as a tumor which starts in the brain (e.g., **glioblastoma**, **astrocytoma**, or **oligodendroglioma**), or as a mass that develops from the coverings of the brain (e.g., **meningioma**). Where the tumor is located in the brain and the brain structures it affects will determine the resulting signs and symptoms. A brain tumor may cause a combination of symptoms, such as cognitive impairment, weakness, and visual loss, with many of the symptoms being quite subtle. Depending on the tumor type, brain tumor–associated dementia differs from most dementias due to neurodegenerative disorders in several ways: (1) it occurs faster, with changes becoming apparent over days or weeks; (2) it may cause neurologic symptoms on one side of the body in combination with the development of dementia; and (3) it may be revealed suddenly by the onset of a **seizure**. Seizures can also occur in people with neurodegenerative dementias such as Alzheimer's disease. Another symptom of a brain tumor is headache, particularly one that worsens when lying down or during activities that cause the person to strain (bending over, lifting, sneezing, straining while using the toilet). When a doctor suspects that dementia is due to a brain tumor, neuroimaging and referral to neurosurgery or neuro-oncology may be scheduled quickly. Since treatment success is more likely when done early in the disease, brain tumors often carry a greater sense of urgency to establish a diagnosis. Another book in this series, *Navigating Life with a Brain Tumor* by Lynne P. Taylor, MD, FAAN; Alyx B. Porter Umphrey, MD; and

Diane Richard (Oxford University Press, 2012), is a useful resource on this topic.

Normal pressure hydrocephalus

Normal pressure hydrocephalus (NPH) is a rare disorder that presents with three primary symptoms—cognitive impairment, urinary **incontinence**, and a specific form of gait disturbance called **magnetic gait** (in which the feet appear to be stuck to the floor when the person tries to walk)—all of which progressively develop over months to years. These clinical findings are tied to a specific pattern on brain imaging (MRI or CT) supporting **hydrocephalus**, an excessive amount of cerebrospinal fluid (CSF) accumulation deep within normal brain structures. This fluid accumulation is not associated with obvious brain atrophy to suggest another cause of dementia, such as Alzheimer's disease. Individually, these symptoms are common with advancing age and may be found in conjunction with many common unrelated conditions. For example, cognitive impairment may be caused by Alzheimer's disease, urinary problems may be associated with prostate or bladder dysfunction, and gait difficulty may result from knee arthritis. However, when these three findings are seen together along with **hydrocephalus** on brain imaging, it is recognized as possible NPH. Hydrocephalus is diagnosed when enlarged ventricles (the fluid-filled spaces in the brain) are seen on imaging. Sometimes as the brain atrophies or shrinks in Alzheimer's disease, the ventricles expand into the extra space, but in the hydrocephalus seen in NPH, enlarged ventricles are present without brain atrophy.

Diagnosing NPH requires a **lumbar puncture (spinal tap)** for CSF analysis (Appendix B). Unique to NPH, the doctor will not just send the CSF to the laboratory for diagnostic tests but will also observe what happens after a fairly large amount of the CSF is removed during the lumbar puncture. If walking or balance show significant improvement after a lumbar puncture, it is suggestive of NPH. An indwelling spinal catheter called a **spinal drain** may be advised after the large-volume lumbar puncture to assist in confirming the diagnosis. A neurosurgeon will place the spinal drain into the lower back in the same site as the lumbar puncture; this procedure requires hospitalization.

The reason a doctor may perform many tests to confirm the diagnosis of NPH is because NPH is treatable by the insertion of a **ventriculoperitoneal shunt** (VPS). Doing so may stop or slow some of the changes in NPH, and in some cases reverse them if caught early. Inserting a VPS is a relatively straightforward neurosurgical procedure but is still major surgery requiring general anesthesia, hospitalization, and a recovery period. The surgery involves placing and connecting a long tube or catheter from the head to the abdomen. The tube is inserted through a hole created in the skull and then passed through the side of frontal lobe of the brain and into the ventricles and connected to a tube running under the skin of the head and chest, so the CSF ultimately drips slowly into the abdomen, where it is easily absorbed (Figure 9.1). Most of the time, a VPS is a one-time procedure, but on rare occasion the shunt can become disconnected or even infected and may need to be replaced. Because insertion of a VPS is neurosurgery, it is not taken lightly by a neurologist, considering the risk of adverse outcomes. The diagnosis of NPH can be challenging, and if NPH is misdiagnosed, the procedure could be performed unnecessarily. However, when the doctor makes the diagnosis of NPH correctly, treatment with a VPS can be life-changing with impressive improvement, especially when the VPS is placed before substantial memory problems emerge.

Brain trauma and dementia

Chronic traumatic encephalopathy (CTE) is a distinct type of dementia associated with repeated head trauma. CTE has caught the attention of the media and public since most people with CTE have been exposed to years of repeated head trauma in various sports with high risk for contact and collision, such as boxing, American football,

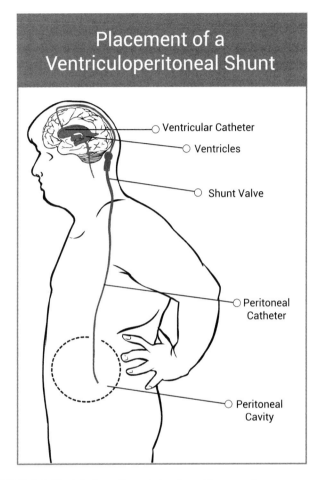

FIGURE 9.1 Ventriculoperitoneal shunt used in normal pressure hydrocephalus. When placing a VPS for NPH, several tubes are inserted into the body and connected to create one long tube that allows CSF to drain from the ventricles deep in the brain into the abdomen outside the stomach and intestines, where the fluid is later absorbed. A shunt valve placed just behind the ear can regulate the rate of flow.

soccer, and hockey. CTE has also been described in association with domestic violence. The clinical syndrome is now called **traumatic encephalopathy syndrome** and may also be referred to by other names, such as **dementia pugilistica**. In older adults, features of the syndrome overlap with features of frontotemporal dementia and Alzheimer's disease, and, in fact, a distinct type of Alzheimer's-like brain change is seen under a microscope. When CTE occurs at younger ages and in middle adulthood, it may be confused with profound depression. The frequency of this disorder in people with sports careers of any length remains unknown. This is an area of active study and has substantial public health implications given the millions of young athletes at risk for recurrent head injury.

Traumatic encephalopathy syndrome is distinct from the common history of a single traumatic brain injury ranging from mild to severe, which may involve a single region of the brain or many brain structures, depending on the injury. Most traumatic brain injuries are not sports related. Traumatic brain injury has been called a silent epidemic since most of the injuries are hard to detect and cannot be seen. Although most people with mild traumatic brain injury have a full recovery, especially those with a single concussion, traumatic brain injury may have substantial effects on cognitive function. In addition to causing cognitive disability, traumatic brain injury may impact family and professional relationships when it occurs in adolescents or young adults transitioning into new family, social, and professional roles. Traumatic brain injury may also occur in someone with a pre-existing cause of dementia. For example, someone with Alzheimer's disease may sustain a brain injury from a fall, and afterward dementia may worsen.

Another complication of late-life brain trauma is the development of a **subdural hematoma**, an accumulation of blood outside of the brain. Typically, this diagnosis is suspected after a noticeable change in cognitive abilities over the course of days to weeks or even months and is discovered on brain imaging. Sometimes those diagnosed with subdural hematomas have a history of a

recent relatively minor head trauma, such as a fall without significant injury or hitting the head in the home (e.g., on a cabinet door),
but often this is not recognized or recalled. Subdural hematomas
can occur on one or both sides of the brain. They are more often
seen in people using blood thinners for medical problems but may
also be identified in people with a history of chronic alcohol abuse,
presumably because of poor balance and chronic risk of falling.
Neurosurgical treatment to drain the fluid or remove the clot is
often necessary but may not always lead to full recovery of cognitive abilities. Resources for support and care for traumatic brain
injury can be found in Appendix C.

Dementia in chronic neurologic disorders

Dementia also occurs in the setting of other chronic neurologic and
psychiatric disorders. About half of all people diagnosed with **multiple sclerosis** have some degree of impaired cognitive abilities at the
time of diagnosis, although these may be subtle. Multiple sclerosis
typically begins in early adulthood and is less commonly diagnosed
in later decades or in those with mainly cognitive symptoms. In severe or treatment-resistant forms of multiple sclerosis, dementia may
develop. In recent years, new disease-modifying therapies have become available for multiple sclerosis. Another book in this series,
Navigating Life with Multiple Sclerosis by Kathleen Costello, MS,
ANP-BC, MSCN; Ben W. Thrower, MD; and Barbara S. Giesser, MD
(Oxford University Press, 2015), discusses cognitive impairment in
multiple sclerosis in further detail.

Other neurologic disorders known as **leukodystrophies** (white
matter disease) affect structures that are involved in multiple sclerosis
but for different reasons and can affect brain functions. Some of these
disorders are caused by how the body and brain clear the byproducts
of our metabolism or handle and store common nutrients in our diet,
such as iron or copper. These disorders are often genetic (inherited)

diseases and often have predominantly young age of onset, with some rare adult forms. Appendix C lists resources on leukodystrophies and metabolism disorders.

Epilepsy is another common chronic condition that affects millions of people worldwide. Seizures are the hallmark of epilepsy and have many different causes, including genetic causes of altered brain function, structural brain changes that occurred in early life, and brain injury in adulthood. Some forms of dementia, such as Alzheimer's disease, stroke, and brain tumor–associated dementia, are associated with increased risk of developing seizures, and some forms of epilepsy are associated with memory changes, especially when seizures begin in the temporal lobe. Many people with epilepsy report some cognitive problems, which are often due to side effects of the medications that treat epilepsy. The cognitive changes in epilepsy are usually not progressive throughout adulthood but may become more obvious in aging when other cognitive disorders emerge and cause dementia. Another book in this series, *Navigating Life with Epilepsy* by David C. Spencer, MD (Oxford University Press, 2016), covers this subject in further detail.

Chronic psychiatric disorders are another category of disease with a clear basis in the brain and are also associated with cognitive changes both in early adulthood and with aging. The most common psychiatric problem, depression, is associated with forgetfulness and executive problems during depressive episodes as well as an increased risk of cognitive impairment and dementia in late life. The scientific basis for this late-life association is not clear. Physicians consider depression as a possible cause for dementia during an initial evaluation, especially when depression is untreated. But it is also true that depression may be a symptom of dementia, especially when present for the first time in late adulthood.

Schizophrenia is a less common psychiatric disorder than depression. Schizophrenia has a connection with dementia, including early onset of an Alzheimer's-like pattern of clinical changes in late life. Schizophrenia affects brain regions associated with memory, including the temporal lobes, and may double the risk of dementia. Resources on depression, schizophrenia, and other psychiatric disorders are listed in Appendix C.

Autoimmune and other acute inflammatory brain diseases

A large number of inflammatory, infectious, and even stroke-like disorders can present as rapidly progressive dementias over the course of days, weeks, or months. The list of these rare potential causes of dementia is long. When cognitive problems develop rapidly, an aggressive evaluation is needed, often while the patient is hospitalized, including an electroencephalogram (EEG), CSF analysis, imaging, and bloodwork looking for antibodies known to cause a rapidly progressive dementia. In some circumstances, acute brain inflammation may occur when the body's immune system unintentionally attacks the brain in response to a trigger elsewhere in the body. This may be in response to an infection or even a cancer. It is important to remember that rapidly progressive dementia may have an identifiable cause and is sometimes treatable and potentially reversible.

CHAPTER 10

Treatment of Cognitive Impairment
and Dementia

In this chapter, you will learn about:

- The medications used to treat cognitive changes in dementia
- The difference between symptom-based treatments and disease-modifying therapies in dementia
- How palliative care is used across all stages of dementia and informs treatment decisions

Establishing a dementia diagnosis can be challenging, and understanding and accepting the diagnosis remain challenging even after the diagnosis is made. Making matters even more difficult, medications that substantially impact the course of dementia for many patients are lacking. Instead, most available medications provide only modest symptomatic relief for the cognitive problems. This chapter describes the pharmacologic (medication) options for the cognitive symptoms of dementia.

All medications used in dementia serve to ameliorate some of the symptoms and potentially improve quality of life. Fundamentally, this is the definition of **palliative care**, which aims to relieve suffering of any kind. Although the term may be used when discussing the end stage of disease, for all diseases, including dementia, palliative care begins the day a doctor makes the diagnosis and begins treatment. Establishing a treatment plan at each visit includes discussion between the person with dementia, the caregiver, and the physician and should cover the following:

- Identifying the primary new, developing, or troublesome signs and symptoms associated with dementia
- Determining what, if any, medications could be considered to address this therapeutic target
- Weighing the benefits of any new treatment against the potential side effects
- Determining if the problem could be addressed more effectively by or jointly with nonpharmacologic strategies

Most medications used in treating dementia help with symptoms of dementia but do not prolong life or delay decline. This begs the question: How can a medication improve symptoms without changing the course of the disease? Understanding this distinction can be difficult, especially when we consider how other common health problems are diagnosed and treated. For example, blood pressure can be easily checked at home or in the doctor's office; if it is consistently high, a diagnosis of hypertension is made and treatment begins. Medications are then adjusted in response to blood pressure changes, and, most of the time, high blood pressure can be managed effectively.

So, why is the treatment of dementia so different than the treatment of other conditions such as high blood pressure? Fundamentally, the most common forms of dementia share the following scenario. Imagine two nerve cells (neurons) sitting side by side that are getting sicker over time because of microscopic neurodegenerative changes. For most persons with dementia, no medications are available to stop those two nerve cells from getting sicker. Instead, most available medications allow the neurotransmitters that connect these two cells to work for a longer period of time (Chapter 4). Without these medications, the neurotransmitters that enable the communication between the two cells would break down more rapidly. The net effect is not just about these two cells; the effects of the medications are multiplied over many nerve cells—perhaps millions or even billions of cells—and the connections those cells make elsewhere in the brain. Unfortunately, the nerve cells continue to get sicker even while the transmitters are stabilized. However, medications that work on neurotransmitters make no real difference to the health or longevity of the nerve cells. This is why all drugs available to treat cognitive symptoms in dementia seem to work for only a little while, from just a few months up to, in some cases, a few years. The problem is most available drugs do not treat the underlying disease that is making the nerve cells get sicker day by day.

As dementia worsens, symptoms change. Sometimes earlier troublesome behavioral symptoms resolve, leading to a phase of disease that is easier to manage. However, as more brain regions are affected by dementia, worse or new symptoms begin to develop and need treatment. As dementia progresses, the medications that once appeared effective may seem to stop working and progressive memory loss again becomes evident. Most likely, the drugs are still doing the job they were designed to do, but because the nerve cells are increasingly injured, the effect of the medications is not as obvious or may have indeed worn off. It is also important to remember that medications may work better in some patients than others for reasons that are not always clear. Several classes of medications that are typically relied upon are discussed later in the chapter.

It is also important to realize that important changes are happening in the field of dementia treatments. We are entering a new phase in which disease-modifying therapies—medications that decelerate biological changes or stop progression—are becoming available. However, at present, there is only one available medication, and it is likely going to be limited to treating those in the earliest stages of Alzheimer's disease, including MCI due to AD. It is expected that other medications may soon follow in treating the underlying biological changes of dementia. With these medications, it is hoped that if some of the underlying brain changes can be stopped or slowed, the symptoms of dementia may slow down or potentially improve.

As is the case in most diseases, the first medications available to treat a disease do not end up being the ones we use years later. But these medications are beginning to provide a path toward better treatment options.

Participating in research is an important consideration for people affected by dementia. It is the only way forward to help the millions affected by dementia. Research may not be accessible to everyone and may depend on where people live or what resources are available for them in order to participate, including study partners. Appendix D discusses research studies and considerations for participation.

Pharmacotherapy: general concepts

Different classes of therapies and medications are prescribed to control specific symptoms of dementia. Regardless of the medications prescribed, a few concepts of pharmacologic management of dementia are important:

- Individual medications can help with some, but not all, dementia symptoms.
- Medications will be selected for use based on the symptoms currently affecting the person with dementia.
- Medications are generally introduced sequentially, allowing for time to pass to determine treatment success or failure. Sometimes variations related to the underlying disease explain the day-to-day changes seen in dementia, rather than changes in medication. Although it is tempting to try several new medications at once, doing so makes it hard to understand what works and what causes side effects. When new symptoms emerge, it can take a few weeks before medications are optimized.
- Timing of dosing can be important. Some medications take effect within an hour of administration, whereas others may not take effect for days or weeks. It is important to understand how quickly medications are expected to begin to reduce

symptoms so you can observe for effects. What you observe will help guide treatment decisions.

• For some symptoms of dementia, no pharmacologic strategies have been approved by the U.S. Food and Drug Administration (FDA), and some therapies are associated with a substantial risk of adverse side effects. Many times, the side effects are acceptable considering the debilitating nature of untreated symptoms.

• When meeting with a new physician, provide a clear timeline of medications used and their observed impact, including side effects.

Therapies in early-stage disease

Treatments for early-stage dementia and MCI can be divided into symptom-based therapies and newly available disease-modifying therapies. At present, there are several symptom-based medications approved by the FDA for treating early-stage Alzheimer's disease, Lewy body dementia, and vascular dementia, but there is only one medication available for treating the biological changes in early-stage Alzheimer's disease (aducanumab).

Disease-modifying treatment for early-stage Alzheimer's disease

Aducanumab (Aduhelm) is the first disease-modifying therapy available for the treatment of Alzheimer's disease in the United States and represents a fundamental change in how Alzheimer's is treated. Instead of just treating symptoms of Alzheimer's disease, it is designed to impact the underlying microscopic or biological changes seen in Alzheimer's disease and, in turn, hopefully slow cognitive decline. The extent of clinical benefit remains uncertain and is likely only modest. It has been approved through a unique accelerated pathway, and its initial availability may be limited.

Aducanumab functions to remove amyloid from the brain, one of the key brain proteins seen in nearly everyone with Alzheimer's disease (see Chapter 5). It belongs to a class of drugs called monoclonal antibodies, which have been used in other diseases but not Alzheimer's disease before now. Monoclonal antibodies use the immune system to fight the biological changes of Alzheimer's disease. Although we may think of the immune system only in terms of how it fights infection, it has been studied extensively and can also be used to treat a range of conditions, now including Alzheimer's disease.

Aducanumab is a once-monthly infusion given under close supervision. Each time an infusion is given, a small intravenous needle and plastic tube (an IV) will need to be placed. The infusion is given over the course of 1 hour, usually under a nurse's supervision. For some other diseases, people receive infusion medications either in infusion centers or sometimes at home, and aducanumab is given in a similar way.

In the studies that led to the medication's approval, all persons had been diagnosed with mild or early-stage Alzheimer's disease including mild cognitive impairment due to Alzheimer's disease. The current indication for treatment with aducanumab is similar. Further, only persons with biologically defined Alzheimer's disease changes will derive any benefit from the medication. Thus, it is expected that many more persons will undergo testing for evidence of brain amyloid based on testing spinal fluid, amyloid PET imaging, or possibly blood tests, which are just now becoming available (see Chapters 2 and 5). Aducanumab is very expensive, and how insurance plans will cover its cost is not yet clear. Everyone treated with aducanumab will need to have an MRI at baseline or within a year of the first dose. Just before the seventh dose (after 6 months of treatment), another MRI will be done, as well as another 6 months later. It is also expected that there may be specific monitoring required for safety and to confirm that the medication works. This will most likely involve standard memory assessments that neurologists routinely do.

Aducanumab is not known to interact with other medications. Other medications used for Alzheimer's disease as well as other diseases can be continued. People taking some blood thinners or who cannot get an MRI may not be eligible to take aducanumab. If a dose of aducanumab is missed, it should be given as quickly as possible. It cannot be given in intervals shorter than 3 weeks apart.

The most common and serious side effects of aducanumab involve areas of brain swelling and even small areas of brain bleeding. These are often detected on MRI brain imaging. Taken together, these changes are called **amyloid-related imaging abnormalities (ARIA)**. ARIA with swelling occurs in about 1 in 3 treated patients, and ARIA with bleeding can occur in about 1 in 5 patients. Most people do not have symptoms from ARIA, but some do. The MRI detects these changes. It is expected that about 1 in 10 patients treated with aducanumab will probably have to stop treatment due to ARIA. Severe symptoms and complications related to ARIA occur in about 1 in 100 treated patients. These and other possible side effects are why specialists, particularly neurologists, are involved in treating patients with aducanumab for Alzheimer's disease. Some people may decide not to take the medication because of these side effects in particular. ARIA is more likely to occur in persons who carry a specific form of the gene apolipoprotein (APOE) called e4. Testing for APOE is not necessary before starting aducanumab. Many patients included in trials were known to carry the APOE e4 allele and were treated anyways. Knowing if you have ApoE4 can help you make decisions about taking the medication, since the risks of complications are higher in persons with ApoE4. Although genetic testing is now easy to get, speak with your doctor before getting tested for ApoE4 or any other gene for Alzheimer's disease or dementia.

Symptom-based treatment for cognitive changes in mild dementia

Since memory loss is the most common symptom in Alzheimer's disease, many studies have been done to investigate medications for this symptom in both early and more advanced Alzheimer's. Most medications studied in those with mild cognitive impairment show that people may be as likely to experience a side effect as a benefit. Thus, it is generally not recommended that medications to aid memory be used in those with mild cognitive impairment.

The standard of care for early stages of some types of dementia is to begin a medication from a class of drugs called **cholinesterase inhibitors**. These medications can help the symptoms of Alzheimer's disease, vascular dementia, and dementia with Lewy bodies but may worsen the symptoms of frontotemporal dementia.

Three cholinesterase inhibitors have been approved (Table 10.1): donepezil, rivastigmine, and galantamine. All are available in a tablet form; rivastigmine is also available as a once-daily patch. In the United States, all are available in generic format and all were first FDA approved for Alzheimer's disease but may have application to a broader range of dementias. Each medication is available in successively higher dosages; whenever possible, the dose is increased gradually to avoid side effects.

Which of these medications is chosen largely depends on your physician's preference and experience. A once-daily medication may be the easiest form to take in any stage of the disease. Although patch formulations of rivastigmine may have the lowest likelihood of

TABLE 10.1 Pharmacotherapies Used in Dementia

	Donepezil (Aricept)	Galantamine (Razadyne)	Rivastigmine (Exelon)	Memantine (Namenda)
FDA approved for	Mild to severe AD	Mild to moderate AD	Mild to severe AD	Moderate to severe AD
Mechanism	Cholinesterase inhibitor	Cholinesterase inhibitor	Cholinesterase inhibitor	NMDA antagonist

The terms mild, moderate, and severe dementia correspond with early-, middle-, and late-stage disease.

producing adverse side effects, many insurance plans do not support using the rivastigmine patch initially and require waiting until oral cholinesterase inhibitors have been tried and poorly tolerated.

For the most part, the three cholinesterase inhibitors are comparable in efficacy and tolerability in persons with mild to moderate dementia. None of these medications provides a clear long-lasting effect on the symptoms of dementia, and it can be hard to appreciate a clear benefit as cognitive decline often continues at some point after the drug is started. It is hard to predict who will benefit from the medications, and some people will respond better than others. Based on many studies, each cholinesterase inhibitor provides some improvement in cognition for a few months, sometimes longer. It is important to understand that the response to a starting dose does not necessarily predict the response to further dose changes. There may be a longer-lasting benefit on caregiver well-being, which is certainly important and must be part of the dementia care equation.

About 1 in 5 treated people will experience some form of side effects, which may occur when cholinesterase inhibitors are started or with any dose increase. Common side effects include stomach upset with nausea, vomiting, or diarrhea. Other side effects include slower heart rate, vivid dreams, or worsening behavior. These medications may also reduce appetite and contribute to weight loss. Many times, the side effects are brief and resolve after several doses, so it's important to be patient. Other times, intolerable side effects such as vomiting may occur every time the medication is taken. When this happens, another medication within the class can be tried. Over time, unintentional weight loss, whether relevant to a medication or not, can become a major problem in dementia and contribute to frailty. Monitoring weight at home can help to minimize the risk of a critical amount of weight loss. Make sure to tell the doctor as soon as any side effects begin.

Sometimes patients are diagnosed with dementia while hospitalized. As tempting as it may be to start medications right away, a hospital stay is rarely the right time to start a cholinesterase inhibitor for dementia as it can be a chaotic time with too many uncertainties. Hospitalization inevitably complicates identifying both the beneficial effects and side effects of new medications. Whenever possible, medications should be started during an uncomplicated phase of dementia to determine what responses are associated with them.

Physicians may have philosophical differences on whether or not to prescribe medications for dementia. Some doctors decide not to use cholinesterase inhibitors because of their relatively modest and brief benefit. They might also be worried about possible side effects. If a doctor chooses not to try any of these medications, there is nothing wrong with asking why, but remember that cholinesterase inhibitors, even in the most appropriately selected patients, often provide a modest but brief benefit and do not change the overall course or duration of the disease or delay transitions in care (e.g., placement in a nursing home or hospice care) or death. Although uncommon, some patients and families describe a significant improvement in cognition or behavior when these medications are used. Even a brief benefit can be worthwhile, especially when quality of life is improved.

In the non-Alzheimer's dementias, the value of cholinesterase medications is less certain as few trials have been conducted to guide practice. Alzheimer's disease and dementia with Lewy bodies have overlapping features, and cholinesterase inhibitors show a similar benefit in dementia associated with Parkinson's disease. In frontotemporal dementia, cholinesterase inhibitors may worsen behavioral problems and thus are often avoided. However, because the side effects are not permanent and some patients have profound memory loss in frontotemporal dementia, they may be tried on a case-by-case basis.

The benefit of cholinesterase inhibitors on other dementia symptoms, including language difficulty, executive function, and visuospatial problems, is not nearly as clear. Because of few alternatives and predictable side effects, cholinesterase inhibitors are prescribed for a range of dementia symptoms.

Treatment of cognitive problems in middle- to late-stage dementia

Although needs may change as dementia progresses, the doctor will use similar principles of care throughout the course of dementia. Medication choices are symptom focused, aiming to decrease suffering. Except for galantamine, all cholinesterase inhibitors are FDA approved for all stages of dementia and are typically continued through much of the course. Aducanumab is not approved for use in those with middle- or late-stage dementia.

Memantine

Memantine is an FDA-approved medication for those with middle- to late-stage Alzheimer's disease. Most trials suggest that memantine is best used as add-on therapy to a cholinesterase inhibitor at a time when daily care needs and disability substantially increase (Chapter 2).

Memantine works differently than the other classes of medications used in dementia in that it blocks a receptor called **N-methyl-D-aspartate** (**NMDA**). NMDA triggers the release of **glutamate**, which is an excitatory neurotransmitter; initially, it was thought that memantine would help by reducing the potentially toxic impact of glutamate in the brain. Despite the promise of this drug's mechanism of action (decreasing a potentially toxic substance in the brain), like the cholinesterase inhibitors, it does not slow disease progression and usually has only a brief and modest impact. However, as with cholinesterase inhibitors, some patients may experience clear improvement in their symptoms for a time. Memantine is available as a generic medication taken twice daily. Brand-name versions of the drug are available in extended-release once-daily formulations that are generally more costly. A combination memantine–donepezil tablet is also available, but this only provides the convenience of taking one pill per day rather than up to three.

Stopping medications for memory in late-stage dementia

At some point in the late stages of disease, it is worth considering the value of continuing dementia medications compared to stopping them. For many, the medications will not have an obvious effect. However, it is possible that medications for memory provide more benefit than is realized. Sometimes, decline is reported by caregivers when memory medications are stopped; it may then be difficult to return to the prior level of function when the medications are restarted. The big question is whether the decline is related to discontinuation of the medication or just the natural course of disease progression. At some point, especially in very late stages of dementia, it may be worth discussing discontinuation of memory medications with your doctor.

Martha is a 93-year-old woman who was diagnosed with Alzheimer's disease 10 years ago. At first, she was treated with donepezil, which she tolerated without any side effects. Four years ago, her husband noticed she was having more memory problems and became unable to pick out her clothes or use the shower. She stopped leaving the house except for doctor's appointments 2 years ago, and earlier this year she became wheelchair dependent and barely talks. Two months ago, her husband died. Martha returns to the doctor with her daughter to review available treatment options. Her daughter wants to take stock of all of her mother's medications and discuss what is essential, including those for managing blood pressure, cholesterol, and memory. After a discussion with the doctor, donepezil and memantine are gradually discontinued. Martha's memory and behavior are not appreciably different afterward, although she is perhaps more tired. Her daughter continues to focus on comfort as Martha transitions to a long-term care facility.

Unproven available treatments

Most physicians can appreciate that patients and families want to find and possibly try anything to help with dementia. Often families search for strategies not approved by the FDA or treatments not routinely considered or recommended by treating physicians. Understandably, families often have a sense of urgency to try anything to help, even if the data driving such decisions are weak. It is important to understand that many unproven therapies are advocated online, with little to no evidence of benefit and the potential for harm. Treatments sought or tried by some families range from pharmacologic treatments, including nutraceuticals (naturally derived products such as coconut oil) and dietary supplements (such as gingko biloba and turmeric), to nonpharmacologic treatments (including hyperbaric oxygen therapy), stem cell infusions, and chelating agents. This list shifts with time, depending on what has caught the collective attention of the public and what is eventually proven unsafe or clearly ineffective. Important considerations before starting a therapy not otherwise recommended include:

- There are no safety data for some over-the-counter therapies when used in dementia, and some natural products may be harmful. Numerous over-the-counter products were once thought to be safe but are now banned after patients with various medical conditions experienced adverse outcomes, including death. Generally these problems only come to light when members of the public who have used these treatments bring them to the attention of the FDA.
- Using unconventional treatment strategies can be costly. In addition to the cost of over-the-counter remedies and holistic therapies, local or international travel to centers to receive these medications may be required. Some opportunists may also charge for treatments that have no basis for use in dementia or even other diseases.

- A potential danger of drug–drug interactions exists, including unknown interactions, between new or unproven therapies and established prescribed medications.

Health care has a long and unfortunate history of improbable cures sold on faith. Many physicians are eager to learn about and prescribe new medications; nearly always, these follow a long road to scientific discovery built on data-driven decisions and closely supervised clinical trials involving well-characterized trial participants. At times, doctors may take a more permissive approach to therapies in later stages of disease when comfort measures become the focus of care, as long as these treatments remain relatively safe. End-of-life care and palliative care are discussed in Chapter 15.

What about stem cells?

The human body starts out as a small single cell that rapidly multiplies into millions of cells, all specialized, from the cells at the base of our fingernails to heart cells to liver cells to brain cells. Yet, despite this single early **progenitor cell** (often more broadly called a **stem cell**), for some reason only brain cells develop the problems associated with dementia. Some studies have attempted to use stem cells to treat forms of dementia, but none of them have proven effective to date. Nonetheless, the idea of replacing injured brain cells with fresh new cells is tantalizing.

Gene therapy

In the past few years, interest in technology and the possibility of developing gene therapies for various diseases has been exploding. **Gene therapy** is a treatment that introduces or alters a gene within the human **DNA** to change the disease course (Chapter 2). In some diseases (including some familial dementias), one gene is responsible for causing the disease, so the idea of focusing on such a singular target to treat the disease is appealing. Major progress has recently been made in treating several single-gene neurologic disorders that were previously thought to be incurable, such as rare muscular and vision disorders.

However, several factors limit the application of gene therapy in the field of dementia: (1) the ethics of introducing or altering genetic material, (2) the relative rarity of the genetic causes of dementia known in dementia thus far, and (3) the challenge of crossing the blood–brain barrier to introduce new genetic material into the brain. We must be able to ensure that gene therapy is selective for the one gene causing the disease and not any other gene, that altering genes in the brain would not affect how other organs in the body work, and that altering the gene in the brain will ultimately treat or prevent dementia. This is an important and active line of research, but gene therapy studies are not currently being performed in dementia.

CHAPTER 11

Treatment of Behavioral and Psychological Symptoms of Dementia

In this chapter, you will learn about:

- The challenges of anticipating and addressing mood disorders, sleep problems, and disruptive behaviors
- Treatment options for sleep disorders in dementia
- How pharmacologic strategies complement lifestyle and nonpharmacologic treatments
- How to anticipate and treat a dementia crisis
- How changes in behavior may reflect new medical problems, including infections

At all stages of dementia, diverse mental health and behavioral symptoms occur. Broadly speaking, these include depression and anxiety; disruptive and even debilitating behavioral changes, including irritability and anger; psychotic features, including hallucinations and delusions; and sleep problems, including delayed sleep onset, irregular or fragmented sleep, excessive daytime sleepiness/napping, and behavioral disorders related to sleep. Collectively, these are termed the **behavioral and psychological symptoms of dementia** (BPSD) or **neuropsychiatric symptoms**. These symptoms can emerge in unpredictable ways and at unpredictable times over days, weeks, or months. Many of these behavioral problems were introduced in Chapter 5 with a timeline of when they may occur in Alzheimer's disease, but given the potential severity of these symptoms, it's worthwhile discussing them in more detail. Figure 11.1 summarizes how these problems are defined and how they may relate to other symptoms.

All people with dementia need a specific, tailored approach to manage BPSD. Finding effective strategies to address each symptom can be challenging. BPSD can occur out of the blue because of progressive brain changes in dementia, but some triggers of behavioral symptoms are predictable, including traveling, moving to a new home, or being in an unfamiliar location. Someone with dementia may quickly forget why they are traveling or moving and where they are going, thus resulting in stress.

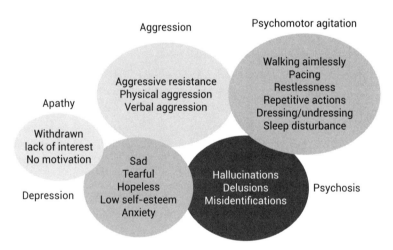

FIGURE 11.1 Summary of behavioral and psychological symptoms of dementia. Depending on the cause of dementia, behavioral and psychological symptoms of dementia (also known as neuropsychiatric symptoms) vary. They can be broadly placed into five categories: aggression, apathy, depression, psychosis, and psychomotor agitation. Characterizing symptoms can help make treatment plans more informed, efficient, and effective.

Source: McShane R. Int Psychogeriatr 2000; 12 (Suppl): 147–153

Richard is an 82-year-old man with moderate dementia. He boards a plane with his partner, headed for home after visiting family on a 5-day trip. The flight lasts for 3 hours, and although he has gotten up to walk and stretch his legs when possible, after 2 hours he is uncomfortable. By the third hour, he is upset and agitated and begins to pace. The final minutes before he exits the plane are unbearable; they are similar to a few other times in the past 6 months when stress made him very upset, such as when he has to bathe. Richard's partner has learned how to help him calm down when he gets anxious, but nothing he tries helps on the flight. As soon as they are in the airport, Richard calms down as if it never happened. Richard's partner later reviews what happened with their neurologist, who suggests a low-dose atypical antipsychotic medication (a tranquilizer) to use on an as-needed basis when the first symptoms of agitation arise.

Mood disorders

Changes in mood are among the more common neuropsychiatric symptoms seen in dementia. While they may not be the most disruptive, they adversely impact quality of life. Fortunately, many patients can be effectively treated.

Depression, apathy, and lack of motivation

The earliest stages of dementia may be mistaken for depression. But in contrast to typical depression in adulthood, which includes the blues, sadness, and tearfulness, depression in dementia is associated with apathy or lack of motivation. Apathy is common in Alzheimer's disease (Chapter 5) and can be particularly stubborn and persistent. Apathy may reflect changes in the brain's reward circuits causing things not to feel rewarding anymore. Or apathy may relate to memory loss: Why read a book when it becomes too hard to remember or upsetting when trying to remember?

It is important to understand that depression in its classic form responds to antidepressants, but the depressive symptoms of dementia often fail to respond. Nonetheless, antidepressants are often tried in dementia and sometimes will help. Sometimes apathy may improve after the patient starts taking a cholinesterase inhibitor, perhaps because of an unexpected primary response to the medication or because improved memory also lifts mood. As with any problems in dementia, apathy and depression in dementia work best ben paired with nonpharmacologic strategies focused on enhancing and expanding activities and daily routines (see Chapter 12).

When a medication is prescribed for depression, the doctor will take into consideration the evidence on its safety and effectiveness, its side-effect profile (which may actually be beneficial for certain mood-related symptoms such as sleep), and their own general experience. Most of the antidepressants provide a similar degree of benefit and vary primarily in terms of side effects.

A key difference between how most antidepressants and the cholinesterase inhibitors act is that antidepressants tend to demonstrate their effect over two time periods. They may start to cause noticeable changes in mood a few days after they are started, followed by more gradual changes over several weeks. Because of this pattern, unless side effects emerge, most antidepressants will be continued for at least 4 to 6 weeks before changes are considered. If the patient has clear depressive symptoms, the response should be obvious: Mood is lifted, sadness improves, and, to some degree, depression is no longer an active or a central problem.

Suicide is a rare cause of death in dementia. Those at risk for suicide include those who have depression early in the course of dementia, along with a tendency to be impulsive or agitated. Those who are aware and able to reflect on their problems and have a means to commit suicide may also be at greatest risk. It is important to discuss any suicidal thoughts or attempts with a physician. Suicide is never the right answer for anyone. Find help and talk to someone if you or someone you know is thinking about suicide. Suicide prevention resources may be found in Appendix C.

When apathy is the main problem, the response to antidepressants may be less obvious, but improvement in engagement and interaction with others may be seen. Although it may seem like antidepressants improve memory, this may reflect improved social engagement or greater ability to concentrate and pay attention because of reduced depression.

Anxiety

Anxiety is another common symptom in dementia. Anxiety includes features of excessive worry, fixation, or obsessiveness over certain things. Anxiety may be more easily recognized by family members than depression as it may be more obvious given the patient's appearance and expression of symptoms, which results in stress for others. When the person with dementia is anxious, caregivers can become exhausted or exasperated. At its worst, anxiety can escalate dramatically. This may occur when the person with dementia becomes aware of the decline in their own cognitive abilities. Uncontrolled anxiety can lead to aggressive or disruptive behaviors.

Your doctor may treat anxiety with antidepressants since these medications are often also effective for anxiety, probably because depression and anxiety involve similar parts of the brain. But antidepressants are not the only medications used for anxiety. It may also be necessary to treat anxiety using medications used for more disruptive and debilitating behavioral problems associated with dementia, including antipsychotics and antianxiety medications.

These medications are discussed further in the section on disruptive behaviors.

Obsessive–compulsive behaviors

Obsessive–compulsive behaviors may emerge in dementia. Examples include obsessive picking, unending cleaning routines, countless trips to the bathroom (unrelated to a bladder problem or urinary tract infection), or being fixated on delusions, which can themselves be upsetting. In frontotemporal dementia, examples of obsessiveness include eating specific, even strange, foods every day or watching a single movie countless times. Much time may be spent checking locks and windows to make sure they are secure. These types of symptoms are very similar to those seen in obsessive–compulsive disorder, which is often first recognized in adolescence or young adulthood. Obsessive–compulsive features tend to respond to antidepressant medications, although higher doses may be necessary.

Intimacy

Dementia may have varied effects on sexual function and intimacy. With anhedonia and depression in dementia, decreased sexual desire may follow. Sexual dysfunction may also be caused by dysfunction of the autonomic nervous system in dementia. At the opposite extreme, **hypersexuality** may emerge, along with other disinhibited behaviors. When delusions occur, the person with dementia may have false beliefs about their relationships. A common delusion is the belief that one's spouse or partner has been unfaithful. Therefore, changes in sexual activity may occur, but intimacy remains a part of the lives of many affected by dementia.

Disruptive behaviors

Among the myriad symptoms that emerge in the setting of dementia, the symptoms that especially challenge a caregiver's stamina, coping skills, and ability to provide care are the disruptive neuropsychiatric symptoms. As discussed in previous chapters, these disruptive symptoms include agitation, irritability, anger, and hallucinations (typically visual and less often auditory). Anger may be accompanied by verbally or physically aggressive behaviors as well as psychotic behavior. Often these episodes occur at the end of the day when the person with dementia is tired, which can worsen confusion. These episodes are called **sundowning**. As the name suggests, sundowning tends to occur in the late afternoon as the sun goes down, when it's time to begin the normal evening routine. Collectively, these disruptive neuropsychiatric symptoms emerge in about one-fourth to one-third of all dementia patients and are particularly problematic in Alzheimer's disease, especially during periods when memory and language decline.

To understand when and why these disruptive behaviors may emerge, consider what a person with memory loss is going through. When everything is confusing, everyone is unfamiliar, and there is no explanation, a reasonable reaction is to become defensive, suspicious, and even aggressive.

Treating disruptive behaviors alleviates suffering

Agitation, anger, and psychosis in dementia are associated with emotional pain and suffering for the patient and caregivers. In deciding on a treatment plan with the doctor, keep in mind the following:

- Few treatments are specifically approved by the U.S. Food and Drug Administration (FDA) for disruptive behaviors in most of the causes of dementia.

- The main class of medications that is often effective in controlling symptoms of psychosis and agitation has an FDA boxed warning stating that antipsychotic medications have been associated with heart attack, stroke, and even death when used by older people.
- Many medications used to treat severe behavioral symptoms increase the risk of parkinsonian symptoms or falls.

The use of antipsychotics and other medication choices can be complex and challenging and should be discussed with an experienced physician to ensure that medications are appropriately selected and monitored. Appropriate treatment options can be determined based on the responses to the following:

- How debilitating are these symptoms when they occur?
- Describe examples of the disruptive symptoms.
- How often do the symptoms occur?
- How do these symptoms impact the person with dementia, the family caregivers, and professional caregivers?
- Do these symptoms disrupt care in some way?

Based on the answers, the physician will consider the risk–benefit ratio (the level of risk compared to the level of benefit) to decide whether medications to reduce disruptive behaviors are needed.

Nonpharmacologic strategies: always the starting point

Reorienting strategies are examples of nonpharmacologic strategies to treat disruptive behaviors. They are nearly always preferable when feasible and are advised in every case, whether or not pharmacologic treatment is required. In the case of disruptive and aggressive behaviors, adaptive strategies to be used in the moment include the following:

- Change or adapt the environment to remove potentially stressful triggers. This may include returning home earlier in the evening rather than staying out late in an unfamiliar place, or even canceling social plans.
- Maintain a supportive tone of voice and demeanor. Proactively describe the current location and date.
- Don't challenge the person's delusions or ability to remember.
- Accept a false memory as the truth and move on, especially if inconsequential. These have been called "fiblets" by some caregivers.
- Try not to enable the person's persistent delusions (e.g., needing to check the bank account repeatedly).
- Try not to lash out when asked the same question many times. Sometimes, writing down answers to commonly asked questions on a card kept nearby can help.
- Change an upsetting subject to another topic or avoid discussing it entirely (such as learning about or recalling a death in the family).
- Use diversions and distractions. Put on some music or the television, create artwork, take a walk, go to the park, go fishing, play with a pet, dance, or do something the person with dementia enjoys but may not have done for a while.

Pharmacologic strategies

When nonpharmacologic strategies are not adequate, medications are necessary for severe, persistent, or threatening symptoms. The first medications a doctor will use to address disruptive behaviors associated with dementia may include the medications used for memory loss, including cholinesterase inhibitors. Additionally, antidepressants, particularly those with some calming or antianxiety properties, may be tried for mild or infrequent debilitating behaviors. However, sometimes the doctor will need to prescribe more potent treatments with a greater risk of side effects. Table 11.1 introduces the

TABLE 11.1 Pharmacologic Treatment Options for Common Behavioral Symptoms of Dementia

Symptom	Treatment options	Side effects	Risks and other notes
Depression and apathy	Antidepressants	Fatigue, confusion, low libido	Apathy is poorly responsive in most people; prescriptive activity plan is often advised along with medication.
Psychosis, agitation, and aggression	Antipsychotics	Fatigue, confusion, weight gain, falls, parkinsonism	Most are not approved for use. FDA boxed warning given risk of heart attack, stroke, and death.
	Benzodiazepines	Fatigue, confusion, weight gain, falls	Do not have FDA boxed warning; can also be used in treating insomnia (see below)
Insomnia	Melatonin	Fatigue	Not an FDA-regulated therapy; brief time window of efficacy
	Antipsychotics	See above	See above; same medication may be used dually as antipsychotic in daytime and to aid with sleep when given in the evening
	Benzodiazepines and other sedative–hypnotics	See above	See above

main groups of medications used for BPSD and the typical conditions for their use.

> *Ernest is a 77-year-old man with moderate Alzheimer's disease. In the past few months, his wife has noticed that he has become short-tempered; he yells at her over the littlest things. Several times he has refused to get out of the car when they go to their daughter's house. He has tried to take the car keys from his wife's hand so he can drive, although he stopped driving 2 years ago when he became unsafe behind the wheel. For the past 4 weeks, he has become increasingly aggressive toward his wife almost every afternoon, and she considered calling the police when it lasted for 2 hours and he threatened her physically. Her attempts to calm him have not worked. After reviewing these recent symptoms with their neurologist and discussing the risks of heart attack, stroke, and even death from the use of antipsychotics, a low dose of the antipsychotic quetiapine is prescribed. Within 2 days of starting the medication, Ernest is much calmer, with episodes of anger lasting only minutes and with less frequency. He is no less confused, but his wife perceives his behavior is better, back to where he was about 2 months ago.*

Which medication and why?

Generally, two categories of medications are used for debilitating agitation, aggression, irritability, paranoid delusions, and hallucinations: **antipsychotics** and **benzodiazepines.** These medications generally do not improve the confusion that contributes to disruptive behaviors; instead, the medications treat the uncontrollable behavioral responses caused by confusion. Measures of success when using these medications include reduced frequency of the symptoms and less intensity of symptoms when they occur.

Antipsychotics

Antipsychotics are classified as "typical" or "atypical," which in addition to their pharmacologic properties largely describes the time period when these medications were discovered as well as their side-effect profiles. Typical antipsychotics were developed long before the atypical antipsychotics and are generally the most potent antipsychotics, but they are associated with more frequent and potentially dangerous side effects. Most of the antipsychotics that have become available in recent years are atypical antipsychotics, which are usually the ones used for disruptive behaviors in dementia. It's important to keep in mind that multiple typical and atypical antipsychotics exist, and finding the best antipsychotic may involve some trial and error. When making a treatment plan that includes antipsychotics, your doctor will consider several points:

- Antipsychotics should be used in close partnership and following a shared understanding between the physician, patient, and caregiver, including recognition of the potential side effects.
- Antipsychotics should be used at the lowest dose and for the shortest period of time, as needed.
- Antipsychotics should be re-evaluated over time with reassessment of the symptoms and side effects.

Neurologically, the most relevant side effects of most antipsychotics include parkinsonian symptoms, such as slowness of gait and other body movements, stiffness, imbalance with increased tendency to fall, and, in some cases, tremor. Some antipsychotics are more likely to cause these side effects, and this may influence which medication is chosen. Parkinsonian symptoms may also be more likely with higher doses of medication used over longer periods of time. Unfortunately, whether or not parkinsonian symptoms occur, when they occur, and to what degree can be hard to predict. Although these symptoms are often treatable and stop once the medication is discontinued, in some cases they may persist even after the medication is removed from the regimen. When this happens, it is possible that the changes seen reflect the natural progression of the disease over time. Pimavanserin is the only FDA approved medication for psychosis, specifically hallucinations and delusions seen in Parkinson's disease. It acts differently than other antipsychotics and is not known to worsen parkinsonism.

Despite the important caveats about risks of antipsychotics, one thing is clear: Appropriately selected antipsychotics definitely relieve the disruptive and debilitating symptoms of dementia in appropriately selected patients.

Benzodiazepines

Benzodiazepines are another class of medications used for some of the same symptoms treated by antipsychotics, particularly anxiety and insomnia. Although they do not have the same side-effect profile as antipsychotics, they are not without side effects, the most common of which is drowsiness. Benzodiazepines are commonly used in many neurologic and psychiatric conditions, and many people are familiar with their use to help control anxiety during airplane travel or other recurring stressors. Benzodiazepines are also prescribed as sleep aids and to relieve muscle spasms. These medications tend to make people groggy and, in some circumstances, forgetful. Although they are helpful given their effective antianxiety and sedating properties, they can cause problems if memory decline outweighs the benefit for agitation and anxiety. More often, they tend to effectively calm the patient. Although parkinsonism does not occur with benzodiazepines, they can lead to problems with coordination, gait, and balance and may increase the risk of falls. Benzodiazepines do not have an FDA boxed warning.

Although it may be appealing to try benzodiazepines or antidepressants first instead of low-dose atypical antipsychotics, antipsychotics may be the better choice since they are generally more effective in controlling disruptive psychiatric symptoms.

Hallucinations, anger, and paranoid delusions that are distressing for the patient and interfere with care tend to respond better to atypical antipsychotics. Anxiety and insomnia may be more responsive to benzodiazepines. Management of dementia is tailored to the individual patient; no two responses are the same, and responses may be unpredictable when new medications are administered.

What time of day is best to administer medications for BPSD?

The timing of each dose of medication used for disruptive behaviors is important to consider. Although every medication works differently, medications used for disruptive behaviors tend to take effect within an hour of administration and tend to provide peak benefit for 4 to 12 hours, depending on the medication. Important points to consider include what time of day disruptive symptoms emerge, whether or not they occur several times each day, and whether the intensity or the type of symptoms differ.

For example, for someone experiencing anger or anxiety as part of late-afternoon or evening sundowning, the timing of the episodes may be predictable and thus treatable. If symptoms begin around 5 PM, a medication can be given around 4 to 4:30 PM in hopes of eliminating or decreasing the likelihood that symptoms will emerge. During the time period when these medications are effective, it may be possible to accomplish tasks such as bathing, which may become difficult because of agitation.

Other treatment options for disruptive behaviors

Several other medications have been suggested to control disruptive behavioral symptoms of dementia, but not much is known about how effective or safe they are. Sometimes medications used as mood stabilizers in other disorders, such as bipolar disorder or severe depression, are tried. These mood-stabilizing medications include valproic acid and lithium. A newer medication that is a combination of two older medications used for other conditions (dextromethorphan for cough and quinidine for leg cramps) has been effective in treating a rare syndrome called **pseudobulbar affect**, which is seen in some forms of frontotemporal dementia. This same medication has been proposed to treat agitation in dementia but may be a less effective option. With increasing social acceptability and availability of marijuana, many families ask about its use in dementia. Several studies are underway to explore if its compounds may help anxiety and agitation in dementia. But there are serious concerns about unpredictable drug levels in marijuana impacting behavior, and potentially worsening symptoms. Until we know more, marijuana is not recommend for use in dementia.

Monitoring behavior after starting new medications

Regardless of which medication is chosen to treat disruptive behaviors, several different outcomes can be expected, and these outcomes will guide the next steps in the management of dementia:

- If the episodes and intensity of disruptive behaviors are markedly improved, the medication choice, dosage, and schedule are likely appropriate.
- If symptoms are somewhat improved but continue, and no side effects are apparent, an increase in medication dosage may be considered or a change in schedule may be warranted.
- If symptoms are improved but improvement is accompanied by fatigue, with frequent napping, the dosage may be too high and/or the medication is being given on an overly aggressive schedule.
- If significant side effects have developed, such as parkinsonism, a change in regimen is warranted irrespective of benefit.
- If the disruptive symptoms are unchanged, either a change in dosage or schedule or a change to a new drug is required.
- If symptoms are noticeably worse or new disruptive symptoms have emerged, a change in medication choice or perhaps even a new class of medication is in order.

Special consideration: dementia with Lewy bodies

Dementia with Lewy bodies deserves special consideration when choosing medications for disruptive behaviors. Paradoxical worsening of confusion may occur with certain antipsychotic medications. Nonetheless, antipsychotic medications relieve the hallucinations and delusions associated with dementia with Lewy bodies and enable the use of antiparkinsonian medications to improve motor function.

Sleep disorders

Sleep disorders are very common in dementia; they can emerge at different times in the course of the disease but may not be a problem for everyone with dementia. Sleep problems in dementia include difficulty with falling asleep, difficulty staying asleep, waking up too early, unusual behaviors while dreaming, and disruptive habits on awakening. Each of these behaviors can be disabling to the patient, bed partner, family members, and professional caregivers. To determine the best treatment for abnormal sleep, the physician may ask the questions in Table 11.2, and knowing the answers will improve the efficiency of managing the problems.

Sometimes it becomes clear that the patient is getting enough sleep, but it occurs at inconvenient times. Fragmented sleep or multiple awakenings may occur but are not necessarily debilitating, especially if they just involve urinating and then returning to bed. Sometimes adjusting the timing of medications or drug choice by the primary care physician can reduce nocturnal trips to the bathroom. Some persons may drink a lot of water, tea, or coffee before bedtime, which may make it harder to sleep and result in arising more often to urinate.

In managing sleep, the doctor may also consider whether daytime behavioral problems in dementia lead to or follow a night of bad sleep. Sometimes insomnia may occur on its own without other symptoms. Determining this can give the doctor guidance in the

TABLE 11.2 Identifying Problems with Sleep in Dementia

Sleep problem	Questions to ask
General	How often does the sleep problem occur? How many nights each week? How many days per month?
Bedtime routine	What is the evening bedtime routine? What activities occur just before bedtime? Do evening meals include caffeine (present in coffee, tea, soda, or chocolate)?
	What else is going on in the home in the evening?
Falling asleep and staying asleep	When is the planned bedtime?
	Does it take the person a while to fall asleep?
	Are there wakeful episodes in the middle of the night?
	What is the morning wake-up time?
Awakening events	What happens with each overnight awakening?
	Does the person go back to bed or start rummaging around the house in the middle of the night? Or begin their morning routine with the intent to leave the house? Or prepare an unsupervised meal?
	How does this impact everyone in the house?
	What dangerous behaviors, if any, have occurred?
Possible evidence of REM sleep disorder	Are there unusual activities during sleep, such as talking during sleep or acting out dreams?
	Does it seem like vivid dreams continue even after waking up?

timing of medications and knowing which symptom should be the focus of treatment.

Sometimes the doctor will refer the patient to a sleep specialist to evaluate the sleep problem more thoroughly and assess for problems with overnight breathing, particularly a problem called **obstructive sleep apnea**, which can impact daytime attention, vigilance, and executive cognitive function independent of dementia. A test called a sleep study (or **polysomnogram**) can also help determine if rapid-eye-movement (REM) sleep behavior disorder is contributing to disturbed sleep. A polysomnogram can be especially helpful for someone who lives alone with no one to witness their nighttime behaviors.

Treating sleep disorders

Medication options for sleep are similar to those discussed earlier for the management of behavioral symptoms associated with dementia because sleep and behavioral problems overlap. These medications may be specifically prescribed to address sleep disorders or prescribed to jointly address sleep, mood, and disruptive behaviors that are pervasive during the day, impact evening routines, and disrupt sleep patterns. Options include antidepressants, antipsychotics, benzodiazepines, and medications that specifically target insomnia.

As may be the case when addressing disruptive behaviors, the doctor may prescribe two classes of medications to be used together—for example, an antidepressant plus either a benzodiazepine or an antipsychotic. Antipsychotics and benzodiazepines are rarely used together because of the risk of more potent side effects.

Zolpidem, eszopiclone, and other sleep aids

Zolpidem and eszopiclone are sleep aids taken by many adults; however, they are not ideal sleep aids in dementia as they can cause excessive fatigue the day after they are taken, even at low doses. These medications can also worsen or cause problems with balance and confusion in dementia. In addition, they are not uniformly successful in controlling insomnia in dementia.

Melatonin

Melatonin is a naturally occurring substance in the brain and is involved in the normal regulation of sleep–wake patterns. It is also available as an over-the-counter sleep aid. Melatonin has been used for many years as a treatment strategy for patients with sleep problems in Alzheimer's disease. Melatonin is used in dosages ranging from 1 mg to 10 mg in most patients and is taken shortly before bedtime. Some persons with insomnia and their families report benefit in sleep quality with melatonin, but it may not be long lasting.

One strategy is to try melatonin when sleep disruption emerges, such as in a pattern of poor sleep several nights in a row. Although the first night may be a missed opportunity, trying it for the next few nights may address the problem. Work with your doctor to determine the length of time to continue to use melatonin. Some prescription medications act at the melatonin receptor in the brain (e.g., ramelteon, tasimelteon), but the effect on sleep problems in dementia may be modest or uncertain. In dementia with Lewy bodies, melatonin may be helpful in controlling the severity and frequency of REM sleep behavior disorder episodes.

Diphenhydramine

Diphenhydramine is an over-the-counter medication marketed under many different trade names and included in many over-the-counter pain medications (typically with a "PM" suffix). It is meant to improve sleep issues in conjunction with common problems such as joint pain, headache, or the common cold. The medication is effective in inducing sleep but has a number of side effects, including possibly worsening the quality of sleep. Sometimes diphenhydramine has a paradoxical effect in those with dementia, causing an increase in energy in the middle of the night and making matters worse. Diphenhydramine may help people fall asleep easily, but they may awaken earlier than expected, causing further distress.

Diphenhydramine is well recognized as a cause of cognitive impairment, and some debate exists about its impact on cognition in older adults when it is taken long term. Given these concerns, the standard practice is generally to discontinue diphenhydramine in people with dementia.

Reviewing the response to medications for sleep

Regardless of the treatment strategy tried, the patient's response to the treatment should be reviewed at each physician visit with the following questions:

- When was the medication taken relative to bedtime? Relative to when the patient fell asleep?
- What is the quality of sleep? If observed, is the person quiet or active while they sleep?
- How did the person feel on the following day? Was there excessive sleepiness?

Responses to these questions will help the doctor determine the next steps. As is the case when optimizing the treatment of disruptive behavior, management decisions are based on patterns of behavior over days or weeks rather than the behavior on a single day or night. Except in the event of a clearly apparent, markedly abnormal response to a newly introduced medication, the pattern of response over longer periods will determine the subsequent treatment course. The following treatment responses may be seen and will guide the next steps:

- If sleeping is much better, and the problem has fully resolved, and daytime wakeful periods continue and may be improved because of improved sleeping, no medication revisions are suggested at this point.
- If sleeping is much better, but the patient has excessive daytime fatigue, and daytime activities are reduced because of fatigue, the medication dose may be too strong or the effect of the

medication lasts too long. A review and adjustment of the treatment regimen is in order.
- If the sleep problems are no better, a review of treatment strategies is warranted.
- If the previously identified sleep problems are getting worse or new ones have emerged, a review and revision of treatment strategies is warranted.

A dementia crisis

This chapter has focused on strategies to address mood, behavior, and sleep disorders in dementia. A rare but well-recognized phenomenon is known as a "dementia crisis," in which symptoms become severe and do not respond to medications. Such a crisis may last for days, resulting in severe distress for the patient and caregiver. Sometimes people with dementia may become aggressive and physically violent. In addition to the challenges of finding the right medications to control severe behavioral episodes, these crises can threaten the safety, well-being, and continued support of personal and professional caregivers.

Sometimes a brief hospitalization is the only way to address acute behavioral problems because treatments only available in a hospital are needed to better take control of symptoms, including physical restraints or medications given by injection when the agitated patient refuses to take pills or pulls out intravenous lines. Unfortunately, staying in a hospital is often very disorienting for a person with dementia since it is an unfamiliar environment with unpredictable schedules that may interfere with sleep. Whenever possible, dementia crises may be best treated in a familiar home environment and in close coordination with the physician. However, it is important to know when to ask for help and when to call 911 if emergency help is needed.

Special consideration: delirium

Delirium is a medical condition characterized by sudden confusion or fatigue that is out of character for the person with dementia, often accompanied by fluctuations in cognitive function and psychotic features, including hallucinations. It usually develops over the course of hours or days. If delirium is suspected, it is important to contact the doctor quickly so that underlying problems, such as a brewing infection (e.g., urinary tract infection or pneumonia), a recent stroke, or new medication side effects, can be addressed quickly. Delirium is a common problem during hospitalization but can occur at any time in the course of dementia. If symptoms of delirium arise shortly after a new medication is started, they may resolve once the new medication is discontinued. Sometimes, however, medications prescribed for disruptive behaviors may help control symptoms, and delirium develops much later in dementia. When this occurs, the likelihood that these symptoms are caused by the medication is much lower, and it is more likely a sign of a new medical problem, warranting the prompt attention of your physician.

CHAPTER 12

Lifestyle Management and Nonpharmacologic Therapies for People with Dementia and Their Caregivers

In this chapter, you will learn about:

- The role of nonpharmacologic therapies in the treatment and prevention of dementia
- The impact of diet and exercise in dementia
- The role of cognitively stimulating and socially engaging activities
- The importance of developing a prescriptive, proactive plan of care
- Methods to support the health and well-being of caregivers

Healthy lifestyle decisions have a potential impact on dementia; they begin with working with your primary care physician to control blood pressure, diabetes, and cholesterol and extend to other preventive health strategies. Any correctable problem, such as visual problems due to cataracts or hearing loss that can be helped with hearing aids, should be addressed, since enhancing the senses can minimize confusion and support memory, as well as enhance engagement with other persons and a patient's environment. Healthy lifestyle decisions may also have a role in either delaying the onset of dementia or slowing its progression in some way.

Once dementia is diagnosed, it is important to consider nonmedication approaches that may help with memory loss. Diet and exercise have the potential to address some of the early brain changes in dementia, but their role in controlling or delaying dementia symptoms remains uncertain. Clearly, regular exercise has many health benefits, including improved flexibility and muscle tone, which may help reduce the risk of falls. Diet and exercise can also help control important stroke risk factors such as high blood pressure and diabetes.

In addition to diet and physical exercise, activities involving socialization and cognitive stimulation may help with aspects of dementia and have overlapping benefits, such as the physical activity involved in leaving the home to attend a social activity. Whether or not these activities impact the underlying disease processes remains a topic of scientific debate.

Some evidence indicates that even after signs and symptoms of dementia have started, **comprehensive lifestyle decisions** focused on diet, exercise, socialization, and cognitive stimulation have the potential to impact the course of disease. For most people, dementia develops and progresses despite appropriate application of lifelong preventive strategies and despite optimizing comprehensive lifestyle decisions once dementia symptoms begin. Some aspects of lifestyle management have no proven bearing on dementia. However, these practices are important in managing the long-term health needs associated with aging, including fighting frailty; maintaining muscle strength, mobility, and balance; and reducing cardiovascular risks. The strategies that are learned, developed, and applied through lifestyle management can have a positive impact on other aspects of care.

Developing a plan of care

Many programs targeting lifestyle management have been developed, including structured daylong programs in local rehabilitation facilities, brief but recurring social programs offered in cultural institutions and through dementia advocacy groups, and individual activities such as online programs. But just as dementia is a highly individualized experience, so is figuring out a plan that works best for you. Consider the following guiding principles when developing a plan that includes comprehensive lifestyle strategies:

- Identify local accessible programs. Some programs are offered virtually and are accessible anywhere.
- Find what works for the person with dementia and caregivers and build on that.
- Brain training games can make people better at the brain training games but have no effect on memory in day-to-day life.
- Try to do as many as possible of the suggested lifestyle strategies; finding success in even one area is better than none.
- Try each program of care a few times. Initial resistance can be overcome after several sessions of an appropriately designed program.
- Start slow, focusing on the easiest problems to fix while forming a strategy to comprehensively target diet, exercise, social engagement, and cognitive stimulation.
- Implement the plan as much as possible, but don't get defeated if things don't go according to plan.

Changes to diet

Some dietary strategies may have relevance to some causes of dementia but likely only before cognitive changes begin (particularly Alzheimer's disease). For most people with dementia, weight stability and a well-balanced diet are the more appropriate, primary goals in diet, focused on sustaining nutrition throughout the course of dementia. Unintentional weight loss is common in dementia, and aside from medication side effects, it is usually related to forgetting to eat or eating only a limited diet, particularly among those without caregivers. Other causes of weight loss in dementia include changes in the perception of fullness or inability to travel to shop at a grocery store.

Weight is an important topic of conversation in any visit with a doctor. Weight control is one of the best-recognized factors in controlling major health problems, including diabetes, hypertension, and high cholesterol, all of which are known to be associated with heart attacks, stroke, kidney disease, certain cancers, and shortened lifespan. But once someone reaches the age of 65, an "obesity paradox" is seen. That is, if someone has lived to this age and remained in otherwise good health, as long as diabetes, high blood pressure, or high cholesterol are not active problems, heavier weight appears to be protective against frailty and bad outcomes after falls. The aging body has a harder time maintaining muscle mass and balance, independent of any disease. Falls become increasingly problematic with age, and, in some circumstances, a fall can be catastrophic and lead to other major problems related to hospitalization for a broken hip, broken shoulder, or brain injury. These injuries can lead to long and difficult courses of rehabilitation and stubborn recovery periods. A higher body mass index (a calculation of weight relative to height) is associated with less frailty, and when a fall happens, less risk exists of some major injuries. However, weight control does not become irrelevant. People with dementia are not advised to gain weight, and any weight-control strategy should also involve monitoring of cholesterol, blood pressure, and blood sugar.

Multiple studies have explored diet and Alzheimer's disease, most of which are focused on the Mediterranean diet. Broadly speaking, the Mediterranean diet includes healthy fruits and vegetables as the source of complex sugars; polyunsaturated oils consumed through nuts and extra-virgin olive oil; and white meats, fish, and legumes (e.g., peas and beans) providing the principal source of protein. For some, small amounts of red wine may be included as part of the diet. Those who have eaten the Mediterranean diet throughout their life may cut their dementia risk by as much as one-third and perhaps much more when coupled with other lifelong healthy strategies, including routine exercise. However, it is unclear whether changing one's diet makes a difference in cognition after one is diagnosed with dementia. It is also unclear why the Mediterranean diet may prevent dementia, but it may have to do with a combination of beneficial effects on the body in general and other healthy lifestyle choices made by those who eat a healthy diet.

Although the benefits of the Mediterranean diet may inspire a move to the Mediterranean isles to prevent dementia (an enjoyable study into which many of us would gladly enroll), eating Mediterranean foods is not necessarily the answer as the diet includes foods that are found in other cultures as well. The Mediterranean diet may also have other health benefits, including lowering the risk of cardiovascular disease and strokes.

Vitamins and other micronutrients found in food

Many research studies in the field of dementia, particularly Alzheimer's disease, have attempted to identify specific components of healthy dietary strategies such as the Mediterranean diet. Areas of the world that appear to have lower rates of dementia have driven some to conclude that specific dietary components or spices must be the explanation for these findings. This compels some people to take a range of supplements. But these differences are now known to be because of the under-recognition of dementia in those geographic areas rather than the effect of any single micronutrient. Across multiple trials, no single vitamin or micronutrient has proven successful in slowing or stopping dementia. In dementia workups, vitamin B_{12} levels are routinely checked and supplemented if low. Beyond this, no consistent evidence exists to support a connection between any vitamin or micronutrient and dementia. Some studies have suggested modest benefits of B-complex vitamins, particularly if patients with dementia have slightly low levels of B vitamins even within the normal range. Taking megadoses of B vitamins is not advised and, aside from cost, can even be harmful.

Alcohol

Alcohol, particularly red wine, has been the subject of research given the potential benefits of the Mediterranean diet. An active compound called resveratrol is found in tiny amounts in red wine and in some fresh fruits and has been proposed as the reason for these potential benefits. Theoretically, some impact on body and brain metabolism may be seen, but the impact of resveratrol on dementia remains uncertain, if any effect exists at all. Moreover, the amount of resveratrol studied in clinical trials is far higher than could possibly be taken through food or alcoholic beverages. Notably, moderate to high intake of alcohol clearly causes memory loss, and some recent studies have even suggested that a low amount of alcohol increases the long-term risk for dementia for some people. Alcohol may also increase the risk of other health problems, including cancer.

Related questions arise about the role of alcohol in dementia care. Many epidemiologic studies have suggested that people who ingest a modest amount of alcohol across adulthood (typically averaging about one drink per day, slightly more for men and less for women) are those with the lowest risk of cardiovascular disease, stroke, and dementia and may be more likely to live longer (in comparison to both heavy drinkers and nondrinkers). However, the role of alcohol in someone with established cognitive impairment is far more complex. Clearly, moderate to heavy alcohol use, termed "excessive" alcohol use, can harm nerve cells in the brain. This damage occurs independent of alcohol dependence or the nutritional deficiencies that often accompany alcohol use disorder. In sum, no studies have shown that alcohol is beneficial for a person with dementia, and in most cases even small amounts may have an adverse impact.

Although the sedative and antianxiety effects of alcohol can be appealing as a home remedy, alcohol use can be counterproductive in the context of Alzheimer's disease by contributing to poor sleep quality, escalating agitation or other disruptive behaviors, and worsening memory. Only in special circumstances should alcohol be used in dementia care, and then only on a limited basis.

Tom is a 68-year-old retired executive who often had several drinks with friends at night. Since being diagnosed with Alzheimer's disease last year, he has been advised to cut back on his drinking, and he has been successful with the help of his wife. But late at night, he sometimes wants a small drink to help him get back to sleep. His wife raises this issue with their neurologist, who weighs the risk of alcohol in the setting of dementia versus Tom's happiness with a small amount of alcohol. Tom's wife notes that when she gives him even a little amount, just a taste really, he often speaks fondly about the friends who used to join him at the social club. And with just a small drink, he calms down and quickly goes back to bed.

Recognizing that old habits die hard, physicians will sometimes encourage drinking less but still permitting a small amount of alcohol on a regular basis. Doing so may satisfy two goals: addressing the issue of excessive alcohol intake while retaining the pleasure derived from having an enjoyable drink. A similar analogy can be made with chocolate, whose antioxidant properties are under study in cognitive aging. Chocolate and caffeine can be associated with agitation if they awaken someone at night. But like Tom's example of having a small drink of alcohol, having a bit of chocolate after awakening in the night may be satisfying and immediately calm behavior. Of course, decisions on whether or not to give alcohol or chocolate, particularly in the middle of the night, must be made on a case-by-case basis, especially if the treat is quickly forgotten after being given. Striking a balance between practicality and goal-oriented behavior, tolerance and prudishness, can go a long way toward ensuring pleasure and happiness. Sometimes it is worth trying something new, as long as it is within the bounds of advisable care goals.

Exercise

Observational, epidemiologic, and interventional studies show the benefits of exercise in dementia, particularly in Alzheimer's disease. Engaging in routine exercise across the lifespan makes one far less likely to develop dementia. Those with regular exercise habits throughout adulthood may cut their risk of dementia by one-third. Exercise also lowers the risk of other medical problems, such as stroke, which impacts dementia risk. Similar to diet, once dementia signs and symptoms begin, the value of starting a new exercise regimen is uncertain. Exercise is also thought to improve attention and mood. As is the case with healthy diet, when included in a comprehensive lifestyle strategy that includes social engagement and cognitive stimulation, exercise may reduce the risk of subsequent cognitive decline in those who are at greatest risk. As always, starting a new exercise routine should be done in consultation with a person's physician to assure it is safe from the standpoint of heart health.

Drawing from these studies, the following general principles are worth considering when planning to include exercise in the management of memory and dementia:

- Any exercise is better than nothing. The goal should not be to run a marathon, but to increase the frequency and duration of physical activities and to engage in new activities whenever possible.
- Determining how, when, and where new physical activities will take place can be challenging at first and may often trigger resistance. Don't give up.
- In addition to starting small, explore the possibility of making physical activities coincidental to the daily routine rather than

a specific activity added to the routine. Walking an extra block or more while shopping is no different than taking a planned walk over the same distance.

- Consider practical limitations, including physical impairments related to stroke, arthritis, or other physical problems related to aging as well as those imposed by the weather. Winter especially makes it difficult to plan for year-round activities.
- If at first you don't succeed, try, try again. However, exercise isn't for everyone, and sometimes pushing the issue may add to stress and interpersonal challenges. As is the case with most recommended best practices, find the way to incorporate physical activity that best works for you.

Socialization and cognitive stimulation

Along with diet and exercise, keeping one's mind engaged, active, and emotionally centered is an important part of dementia care. Exercise, socialization, and cognitive stimulation are associated with a "use it or lose it" concept, and the theory of cognitive reserve (Chapter 5) closely aligns with levels of socialization and cognitive stimulation. Individuals with high cognitive reserve are typically those who not only received more education when young but also continue to keep themselves socially engaged and cognitively stimulated across the lifespan.

Some activities are rich in both socialization and cognitive stimulation. Socialization refers to the act of connecting with someone during or after an enriching activity. These activities may occur naturally and regularly as part of a weekly or daily routine, such as a trip to a local hardware store or barbershop, encountering neighbors during a walk in the neighborhood, family gatherings, or weekly visits to a house of worship. Cooking can be a socially engaging and naturally recurring activity for most. Sometimes the family matriarch or patriarch known for being the family chef develops dementia. They can be kept engaged in cooking when family or caregivers are involved with meal preparation (e.g., by washing or cutting vegetables) while more challenging or risky aspects of cooking, such as using the stove top or range or following the recipe, are eliminated. Cooking may allow the person with dementia to continue a long-standing role that may be part of their identity. As life increasingly moves online, connecting with friends and family through virtual calls or phone calls can be another form of socialization.

Cognitively stimulating activities engage multiple brain functions, including attention and concentration, executive abilities, language, memory, and visuospatial skills. No clear evidence suggests that any one type of cognitive activity is better than another. The most important aspect may be whether the activity can be accomplished and enjoyed and is sought out time and again. Just as an idealized but unpalatable diet will quickly grow tiresome, some activities may not be worth the time or effort invested.

Cognitive activities may be helpful in dementia for a number of reasons:

- Stimulating brain regions associated with the activity as well as a network of related brain structures and circuits
- Using brain regions that are less affected by dementia to help other brain regions that are more affected
- Facilitating social interaction or physical exercise that occurs coincidentally with the planned cognitive activity

Caregivers may also learn to adapt strategies learned during cognitive activities to other circumstances.

Identifying opportunities to connect cognitively stimulating activities with socialization can be especially fruitful in addressing several needs at once. A wide range of cognitively stimulating activities have been proposed and used in dementia care, and some are more well studied than others. These activities range from intense cognitive training with minimal social engagement (e.g., computer-based cognitive training exercises) to activities with strong social connections and little cognitive demand (e.g., a social hour after a religious service), with activities between the two that provide both cognitive and social engagement. Some activities may provide additional emotional support for caregivers and care partners. For example, shared arts-centered experiences coordinated with local art museums (Figure 12.1) can incorporate social interaction, reminiscence, and emotional connections to the material viewed or created, often done with the others involved in the activity. Similarly, playing or singing music can offer a shared social experience and kindle autobiographical associations. Watching television or movies can be considered "cognitive leisure" if enjoyed with others, particularly if it involves conversation and reminiscence.

The optimal cognitively stimulating and/or socially engaging activity will be tailored to the individual, building on preexisting interests or activities. People with dementia often return to activities they had set aside in adulthood. For example, if someone sang in the school choir but didn't have opportunities to sing during a busy working life, they may take it up again in retirement or after a diagnosis of dementia, or a passionate art student who pursued an unrelated career may return to drawing and painting after retiring because

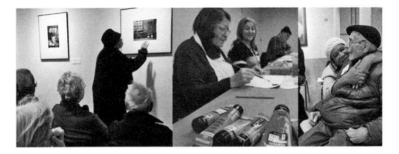

FIGURE 12.1 **Social programs at a local museum.** One social activity for people with dementia that is available in some areas and online involves observing, describing, and creating art. Social and emotional connections are commonly made in these low-risk, rewarding activities.

of dementia. Try to occupy as much of the day as possible with meaningful activities.

Regardless of the activity, one of the hardest parts is getting started, and once activities are designed and planned, they might not succeed despite best efforts. It is hoped that the person with dementia will accept planned activities, but often resistance and even refusal can occur. In many cases, once an activity is attended at least once, there may be greater willingness to attend thereafter. Although people may have substantial limitations in memory because of dementia, emotional familiarity often develops after several sessions when participating in an enjoyable activity in a welcoming environment. Success with one activity may enable others. Try to set a goal to get out of the home every day of the week, making this part of the normal daily routine. A weekly Monday trip to the local senior center for low-impact activities or the art museum can lead to Tuesday's trip to the bakery, Wednesday's trip to the grocery store, Thursday's walk to the park, and so forth. Take notice of surroundings and talk about what is seen, heard, smelled, and felt (e.g., the changing leaves on the trees in the park, the sounds of children playing, the scent of freshly cut grass, the warmth of the sun on your skin). Tapping into the senses can deepen the enjoyment for everyone. Many families find that once these activities are tried, they become increasingly enjoyable and part of the normal routine.

CHAPTER 13

Dementia Care Support

In this chapter, you will learn about:

- The differences between personal and professional caregivers
- How to find a dementia care professional and other resources
- Strategies to effectively introduce a professional caregiver into care delivered at home
- The importance of supporting the needs of dementia caregivers
- The resources for care available as dementia progresses

Caregiving for people with dementia can be an intense and stressful but rewarding experience. Identifying care plans and resources to help support caregivers and care partners is important so that timely, efficient, and effective care can be delivered. Caregivers and care partners may be spouses, children, grandchildren, or close friends. Professional caregivers can help with a range of needs, often depending on the stage of dementia (Chapter 3).

Caring for people with dementia is incredibly time-consuming. In dementia, the duration of caregiving is often longer and greater emotional stress is felt by caregivers than with other chronic medical diseases, such as cancer or heart failure. Thus, ensuring support and care of the caregiver can be just as important as ensuring support of the person with dementia. Depending on the caregiver's phase of life, the availability of material support and resources, and the individual patient's stage and needs, care may be delivered through a combination of personal and professional caregivers over the course of dementia.

Professional caregivers may be hired to serve a specific role or set of roles (e.g., companionship during excursions, home safety monitoring, or advanced/skilled medical needs), perform certain tasks (e.g., simple house cleaning, cooking and meal preparation), or provide respite for family caregivers who need to spend some time outside the home. Local statutes may preclude professional caregivers from coordinating medications or dispensing them but may allow them to provide reminders when medications are due. Depending on the patient's insurance, the cost of a professional caregiver may be covered or may need to be paid with personal funds. Some insurance policies permit family members to be paid for serving as caregivers as a means to offset their loss of income.

Finding a professional caregiver

Professional caregivers are usually identified by referral to an agency providing services or when family members directly contact professional care agencies. Referrals for home needs assessments are initiated by either a physician or a family member seeking additional services. The referral may highlight the following concerns:

- Home safety, such as risk of falls, cooking safety, and medication supervision, particularly during times when the patient is alone
- Skilled nursing needs, such as delivery of injections (e.g., insulin for diabetics), wound care, or instruction in how to use medical assistive devices
- Unskilled needs, such as care coordination to ensure appointments are kept, shopping, cooking, housecleaning, or coordination of other daily tasks

Once a set of needs is identified by a referring doctor or evaluation from a home care agency, the request is submitted to the insurance company or provided to the family member who may be paying for the services. Many families will directly contact home care agencies to provide support during times of need with specific expectations determined at that time; this approach may offer more timely services but may not be as effective.

Some states have training programs to improve the skills of local professional caregivers and provide certification. Many families are interested in finding a professional caregiver who has a cultural background similar to the patient or a shared language, but this may not always be possible. In addition to referrals through professional agencies and physicians (including those working directly with a social worker), dementia advocacy groups are often able to link patients and families to caregiver services, including hospice care. A list of some available services is provided in Appendix C. Many advocacy groups listed provide information about available resources, including those locally available. It may be possible to find a reputable caregiver by asking fellow members of a house of worship, because others may be going through similar challenges. Professional independent geriatric care coordinators can also help identify caregivers and contend with the challenging social situations associated with dementia; however, they can be costly and difficult to find.

Introducing a professional caregiver

Introducing the new caregiver into the dementia care equation can be tricky; it may undo a significant amount of progress made by family caregivers and serve as an unrecognized stressor. Challenges may emerge when introducing a new caregiver for the first time, but some can be anticipated and addressed. Because some people with dementia will resist unfamiliar people serving as professional caregivers, the introduction of caregivers should be done in a patient-centered manner:

- Introduce a new caregiver gradually and with a family caregiver present. Plan to have overlapping periods of time with both family and professional caregiver, with increasingly less overlap over several days. Family caregivers should plan to leave for only brief excursions at first and gradually build up time away.
- Patients with dementia can become familiar with and trusting of new people, although they may not remember their names. This may be more likely when the process and tips suggested are used.
- If the introduction of a new caregiver leads to agitation or aggression in the person with dementia, adding new medications for behavior may help.

Above all, be patient, try again if necessary, and stay in contact with your doctor or local dementia support and advocacy organization to help implement a caregiver plan.

Care of the caregiver

Support from caregivers is essential for patients with dementia throughout the course of the disease. Caregivers face a range of challenges with both physical and emotional stressors, and their needs change over the course of the disease.

Dementia can be painful for family caregivers at all stages of the disease and even after the person with dementia dies. One of the greatest challenges faced by many family caregivers occurs in later disease stages when they are not recognized by the person with dementia or are called by someone else's name. Patients with dementia cannot recognize others or express themselves properly because of the disease. As they slip back into their past and recent memories are lost, the memory that their children have grown and their spouses have aged will also be lost. Patients may perceive that they are living at an earlier time in their life when their children were not yet born or had not grown into adulthood. However, no matter whether a family caregiver is recognized or forgotten in advanced dementia, a familiar, trusted, and loving relationship can continue.

Providing care for someone with dementia is hard. Although it helps to have a realistic picture of what lies ahead, it is also necessary to find a positive path through the disease's darkest moments. To optimize the health and well-being of the caregiver, it is important to remember the following:

- There is more than just sadness in dementia. Try to find humor and sources of well-being in everyday life.
- Try not to get angry at the person. It is the disease talking and acting out, not them. It can be easy to lose sight of this.
- Love the person with dementia. Remember them for the important role they have in your life.
- The caregiver serves as the glue in the caregiver–patient relationship. Without the caregiver or when the caregiver's physical, mental, or spiritual health suffers, a system of care can fall apart. Caregivers need time to prioritize their own needs, including addressing their own medical problems.
- The course of dementia is often long; in some cases, the person with dementia outlives the caregiver. It's important to develop a backup plan to care for the person with dementia.
- Caregivers need to find time for themselves, so they should ask for help.
- Find a way to connect with a loved one with dementia, bringing parts of their past into the present, such as hobbies, activities, and old memories.

Escalating levels of care: it's OK to say "enough is enough"

Despite the best efforts of families and professional caregivers to keep persons with dementia in a comfortable home environment, many will require some degree of coordinated or supervised living in a local facility or institution. Tipping points, or events that lead to a transition of residence for the patient, differ from family to family. Most transitions in care are triggered by one or more of the following:

- Primary family caregiver burnout, illness, frailty, or death
- Inadequate personal or professional resources, regardless of dementia stage
- Changing needs of the person with dementia following acute hospitalization for related or unrelated problems
- Medically refractory and severe behavioral problems
- Apathy and personality changes
- Challenging urinary or stool habits not sufficiently addressed by adult diapers and regular bathroom schedules
- The need for end-of-life care and hospice (Chapter 15)

No two families are alike, and any reason to ask for help (including institutional care) needs to be discussed fully. Asking for help will serve the best interests of the person with dementia and may provide comfort and alleviate suffering. Although later stages of care are often the most costly, they may actually be affordable (Chapter 15).

Day programs

Care provided outside the home can largely be divided into two categories: day programs and residential living. Geriatric social **day programs** are typically programs offered in local centers that may be independent or affiliated with a nonprofit organization, religious group, care facility, or even museum. These programs fulfill an important role in dementia care by offering activities that include socialization, cognitive stimulation, and modest physical activity (Chapter 12). No two programs are alike; some may be more or less sophisticated, culturally tailored, or appropriate to your loved one, and they may have variable costs.

Social day programs offer a variety of activities in terms of frequency and duration and may be tailored for certain stages of disease. Some day programs are geared toward the earliest stages of memory loss, and most day programs are structured so that patients can attend alone to provide periods of respite for family caregivers. However, some community-based programs, particularly those in museums or engaging the arts by other means, include joint participation of the patient and either personal or professional caregivers. Participating in these programs jointly as caregivers and people with dementia can encourage similar and other new activities in the home.

Residential facilities and institutions

Transitioning a patient to around-the-clock care in a residential facility is a difficult process. Residential facilities have several names that are often inconsistently applied, including **independent living**, **assisted living**, residential care, **subacute nursing facility**, memory care, and **nursing home**. When considering transitioning a patient to a long-term care facility, consider the following:

- What programs and resources are offered in the facility? On what schedule are they offered? What is the ratio of instructors to participants?
- Do the resources offered match the patient's needs? Are they a good match with the patient's lifelong habits and preferences?
- Geography matters. Is it hard to get to the facility for visits?
- Whenever possible, visit and tour several candidate facilities. What impressions did you get about the facility in general?
- What is the cost of the facility? The length of time spent in these facilities can be long but is often unpredictable. Costs may also vary dramatically from one region to another.

- Facility metrics indicating measures of quality are increasingly being developed and published online, following a number of governmental mandates. Medicare provides public ratings of nursing homes in local areas.
- Facilities vary in terms of whether medical care is coordinated and delivered onsite or offsite. Are the patient's medical needs likely to be easily met by the facility?
- Do the potential benefits of moving the patient from the home outweigh the potential risks? Does a decision to move fit with the patient's preferences? From a "big picture" perspective, is a move in the patient's best interest even if they previously stated they preferred to live at home?

Generally, the levels of care exist on a continuum. An independent living facility is a good fit for someone who is living independently in the community but needs to move into a coordinated facility for one of the reasons covered earlier this chapter. Independent living may include services such as assistance with bill paying, medication management, social activities, and meals. **Assisted living** facilities typically offer more services, including medication administration and some nursing assistance. **Nursing homes** (which may be called by other terms such as residential living) usually offer an escalating number of services that can be tailored to the needs of the patient. Many assisted living facilities and nursing homes offer memory care services, and many nursing homes also offer hospice care. Subacute nursing care, also known as transitional care, may be provided in the same facility as a nursing home but typically has a finite time window of care anticipated (e.g., the recovery period following the initial hospitalization for stroke).

Take-home point

Find the residential facility that best fits everyone's needs in terms of services, quality of care, convenience, support, and cost.

CHAPTER 14

Monitoring and Maintaining Independence, Safety, and Mobility

In this chapter, you will learn about:

- The importance of identifying and understanding issues of independence, safety, and mobility
- How to support independence through coordination of medications and bills
- How to develop a comprehensive safety plan focused on reducing the risk of accidents and injuries
- How to work through challenging situations, including when employment should end or when driving needs to stop
- Assistive devices and technology that can help maintain safety, mobility, and independence in the home and help caregivers

Broadly speaking, approaches and tools that can enhance dementia care focus on three main issues: independence, safety, and mobility. In the same way that phones and computers enrich and support our lives, assistive devices and technologies enrich and support dementia care, and, as with phones and computers, no single device or approach answers all dementia care needs. Instead, it is important to consider what needs are faced at each stage of dementia (Chapter 3) or may be forthcoming and how to successfully address and anticipate them.

Maintaining and supporting independence

Maintaining independence is a central goal at the beginning of the course of dementia. This section discusses how to avoid financial risks and transition to shared responsibilities in managing bills, practical considerations when employment is affected by cognitive decline, and when and how to address concerns with driving, which is one of the most challenging issues in dementia.

Bills, banking, and taxes

In dementia, cognitive problems can impact the skills required to pay bills, manage banking, and prepare annual tax returns. For nearly all people with dementia, someone will eventually need to take over responsibility for bills and financial organization. Anticipating needs as far in advance as possible is important to avoid problems faced when bills are not paid. Specific financial needs in dementia include the following:

- Scheduling payment of bills
- Establishing shared access to online banking information with a responsible individual
- Taking steps to avoid being taken advantage of by scam phone calls seeking financial information
- Safeguarding essential documents and wallet contents (e.g., driver's license and credit cards)

The need for assistance with managing financial affairs often gradually becomes apparent over time and coincides with gradual cognitive decline. One of the greatest challenges families face is realizing that help is needed, especially when the dementia diagnosis is delayed. Sometimes, the need for help with bills and banking can arise suddenly, such as when a person with dementia faces the death of a spouse who was previously responsible for the bills.

Several options exist for co-management of banking and bills, including establishing a co-signer or having a joint account. The various roles should be set up in conjunction with an experienced elder care lawyer or personal tax attorney to help minimize personal financial risk. Creating either shared access to or responsibility for accounts allows for observation to ensure timely payment of bills while affirming a person's sense of independence. Loss can be limited through real-time fraud notification, which is available through many credit card vendors. Fraud-notification programs often provide a cap for charges and send a message to an account holder when a charge exceeds that amount or for other suspicious activity. People can also be provided with a prefilled debit card with an amount acceptable for loss if the card is misplaced. These strategies allow patients to feel that they are still capable of making banking decisions and purchases.

Employment

Participation in cognitively stimulating and socially engaging activities may benefit people with cognitive impairment (Chapter 12). Employment often meets both needs, given the innate social engagement, familiar environment, and cognitive stimulation associated with work. When to stop working can be a challenging decision for many reasons, ranging from financial implications to social opportunities and friendships. Stopping work is often a clear indicator that real cognitive changes have started. The decision to stop working can be very stressful and poses a risk for an episode of depression in people aware of their ongoing cognitive changes.

However, for some people, stopping work can unexpectedly allow for new cognitively stimulating and socially engaging activities and hobbies to begin or allow them to become re-engaged in old hobbies. Work can sometimes be an ongoing reminder of cognitive impairment when brief or subtle episodes of memory impairment can be personally upsetting, particularly for those with cognitively demanding jobs and especially if others at work notice. For some professions, continuing to work when cognitively impaired may be unsafe and may have implications or repercussions on the health or financial well-being of the patient or others. This may be particularly relevant to health professionals, attorneys, and some consultants, depending on their roles, expectations, and responsibilities. Some people may have little supervision from others, and it can be difficult to determine whether it remains safe to work. Decisions to continue or end employment must be made on a case-by-case basis, with involvement of those affected by the decision whenever possible.

Driving

Driving a car is a clear symbol of independence for many, providing the freedom to go anywhere at any time. Driving is also a routine daily activity that is adversely affected early in the course of dementia, and the ability to drive can be difficult to determine in a physician's office. However, continuing to drive may pose a substantial risk to not only the health and safety of the person with dementia but also that of the public. Driving is an incredibly complex activity that most of us take for granted every day: It requires recollection of a planned destination, working knowledge of a complex map, the ability to see and understand an ever-changing chaotic environment, and the ability to move hands and feet quickly in response. Whether it's in the countryside or on the streets of Manhattan, driving can be dangerous.

For many, a natural movement away from driving occurs with aging, beginning with less distance driving and more local driving. It is well established that cognitive impairment affects driving abilities, most often becoming noticeable in people with mild dementia and sometimes in those with mild cognitive impairment. For nearly every person with dementia, driving must stop at some point, and deciding when is one of the most difficult discussions. Assessing the person's driving safety and preparing for the loss of driving privileges should be done as early in the course of illness as possible, and reassessment should occur on a regular basis. Most states only require basic information and visual acuity to renew a driver's license. Predicting who can drive well and who cannot by assessing cognition in the physician's office is difficult, but factors that can help determine whether driving is potentially unsafe include the following:

- A low score on office-based memory testing or indicators of increasing difficulty with accomplishing normal day-to-day activities
- Perception of the driver's safety by a reliable caregiver who often accompanies the patient as a passenger. If a family member or care partner has avoided being a passenger in a car driven by the patient, was it because of concern for safety?
- Review of the patient's driving record, including minor accidents, tickets, and unexplained dents and scratches. Small dings on a bumper are common and may not be the driver's fault, but scrapes or larger dents are more concerning.
- Multiple accidents and severe cognitive impairment. These are the clearest indicators for a physician to determine that driving is unsafe.

Based on this information, the doctor may initiate referral for an independent driving evaluation or decide that driving should stop immediately. In most places, driving evaluations are not done through a state agency but instead by a physical therapist in a physical rehabilitation center, often in conjunction with a local driving school. Driving assessments are composed of two separate tests: a test of knowledge of the rules of the road with a brief memory assessment and a behind-the-wheel assessment or simulated virtual evaluation. A real in-car assessment is often preferred; otherwise the patient may discredit the results because of the unfamiliar nature of a virtual or simulated assessment. These evaluations usually cost several hundred dollars; some, but not all, insurance policies may cover the evaluation.

After a formal driving assessment is completed, one of several formal determinations is made:

- Safe to continue driving; no remediation is necessary
- Safe to continue driving, but some remediation is recommended to address minor problems
- Unsafe to drive but skills may improve with training; a driving skills course can be tried, but driving is not allowed until proven successful
- Unsafe to drive and skills will not improve; no remediation plan is recommended

For a person who is deemed safe to drive, usually the plan is to monitor the person with a repeat driving evaluation on a regular basis, perhaps annually; however, this should be dictated by monitoring signs and symptoms of cognitive impairment through caregivers on an ongoing basis (including by riding as a passenger) and periodic physician visits.

When driving is deemed unsafe, driving must stop immediately. Although it may be tempting to help or permit someone with dementia to drive, significant public health and legal problems can result from doing so. Being unfit to drive because of dementia can cause the same type of driving errors as those made by a badly intoxicated driver. Impaired drivers risk not only their own safety but also the safety of others. Unfortunately, many serious accidents are caused by cognitively impaired drivers annually, resulting in harm to the drivers and others. When discussing the need to stop driving, the person with dementia often feels wrongfully accused and may take it as a challenge to an otherwise safe lifelong driving record. An effective tactic is to reaffirm a solid driving record and state that stopping driving does not change that. Many people worry about losing their independence when driving ends, so it is important to reframe the discussion to emphasize that drastic changes in independence can result if a car accident causes an injury. It can also be helpful to shift blame for driving restrictions from a family member to the doctor.

In many states, physicians are obligated to report unsafe driving for any reason to the state's Department of Motor Vehicles. Although this is an important formality, whenever possible, the subject of driving cessation should begin well before this determination has been made and well before referral for a driving evaluation. The physician may be put in a position of opening the discussion for the first time, although clear signs of impaired driving may have been recognized by others, including law enforcement. In rare circumstances, a person with dementia may be very upset when driving is restricted and threaten to continue driving. More direct measures may be necessary, including taking away car keys or even the car. Several general principles can help lessen the blow when communicating the need to stop driving:

- Start the discussion early, and not just with the physician.
- Establish a shared commitment to follow the recommendations of an independent driving evaluation before it is conducted. Reinforce this, and consider even getting the patient to write out, sign, and date the commitment.
- Focus on the goals and destinations of car travel. Driving is just a means to a certain end. Do whatever is possible to ensure as little disruption in the person's normal daily or weekly routine as possible.
- Identify options for replacing driving, including rides provided by friends or family members.
- Use supportive language and terms when discussing driving issues whenever possible.
- Refer to the clear data-driven decision provided by an independent driving evaluation.
- Deflect anger or resentment by the patient away from friends and family members who made the determination that a driving assessment was necessary.

Gun safety

Some hobbies may pose unexpected risks if complicated routines are not followed. These can include a range of activities such as scuba diving or skydiving, but the hobbies with potential risks that are most common in the United States involve the use of guns. For many people, guns, hunting, and even teaching gun safety can be lifelong passions or hobbies strongly bound to an individual's identity. The deep connection to guns can be analogous to driving, including the sense of independence and pleasure.

Discussions about the use and safety of guns in the context of dementia can be very challenging but are always necessary. Handling guns requires following well-defined rules of safety, including knowing when a gun is loaded, uniformly following a safety protocol such as keeping the safety on at all times until just before firing a shot, and appropriate directional pointing of a gun. Clearly, each of these steps can be impacted by cognitive impairment. Although uncommon, gun safety assessments can be conducted if a person remains passionately interested in maintaining a gun or hunting hobby. Decisions about continuing to use guns can be considered based on this assessment in a similar manner to basing driving decisions on driving assessments. It is important to discuss gun use with a physician as early as possible in the course of dementia. As is the case with many challenging scenarios in dementia, setting a supportive tone is always ideal, and involving the person in a supportive way is essential.

Sometimes it is possible for people affected by dementia to remain engaged in the social fabric of hunting without handling guns themselves. Hunters may recognize the social connectedness of the experience of hunting and weapon cleaning and maintenance. The act of actually firing the weapon may be the least meaningful part of hunting. Persons with dementia may accept the need to give up shooting a gun as long as the social aspects of hunting can continue. As is the case with impaired driving, catastrophic events connected with gun use can occur at unexpected times, but, when appropriately framed, risk scenarios can be anticipated and minimized. The same holds true for any hobby associated with potentially catastrophic risk caused by carelessness due to cognitive impairment.

Enhancing safety and reducing catastrophic risks

Safety concerns and risks are some of the most important aspects of dementia care but can be among the hardest to recognize and address. A primary goal is to anticipate and avoid catastrophic events related to dementia. Whenever possible, putting plans into place early in the course of illness is an ideal approach to eliminate such risk. This can have benefits beyond personal safety for the person by also minimizing worry. When developing safety plans, it is important to thoughtfully anticipate potential risks and identify the times and situations where the person with dementia is most vulnerable.

The most worrisome and potentially catastrophic events that occur in the course of dementia usually occur with moderate dementia or in middle-stage disease (Chapter 3) when the person with dementia still has some mobility but has increasing confusion and may have emerging problems not yet recognized. Serious events include wandering, accidental kitchen fires, medication errors, and falls. These events may occur when the person with dementia is unaccompanied or unwitnessed, so minimizing the time that the person with dementia spends unaccompanied may prevent these problems from happening or allow help to be quickly provided when they occur.

Wandering

Unfortunately, many people with dementia will wander away from their families or out of their homes at unexpected times. Wandering is associated with major risks of falls and injury and with caregiver distress when the patient cannot be located. Wandering can lead to exposure to the elements in extreme summer or winter weather conditions, falling, or injuries due to carelessness, such as crossing a street when a car is coming or against traffic signals. Leaving the home without notice or leaving a caregiver's side is not done intentionally: The person may be falling into a previous daily routine or reacting to a momentary curiosity. Families are often reconnected relatively quickly based on the person's expected habits, such as visiting a favorite store in the neighborhood. However, when the person is in an unfamiliar environment, tracking them down may be much more difficult. Often, people with dementia do not know that they are lost or that others are expecting them.

Two approaches can reduce the risks and complications of wandering and getting lost: preventing wandering in the first place and finding the person who has wandered off. Prevention begins by anticipating or recognizing times that lead to wandering. Wandering is most likely to occur when someone is alone but may even occur when responsible carers are present in the home. For example, after awakening in the middle of the night, someone with dementia may go through their previous normal adult morning routine (e.g., preparing for a job from which they have long since retired) and then exit the home, unheard by family caregivers sleeping in another room. Building codes typically require keyless locks be used on the interior side of the door in case of fires or other emergencies requiring quick exit. Several models of special keyless, tamper-resistant locks exist that are very effective in preventing wandering, because it can be hard for someone with dementia to figure out how to use them and open the door. Of course, this requires someone else be with them inside at all times in case of an emergency such as a fire. Door and window alarms can alert caregivers of an unexpected opening.

Proactive plans can facilitate the recovery of a person when they wander away from a caregiver in busy settings, such as a crowded street fair. The two broad categories of recovery strategies are low-tech and high-tech solutions. Low-tech solutions include a simple medical information bracelet, pendant, or watch that states the patient's name, diagnosis, and important contact information. A number of local and national programs (e.g., the Alzheimer's Association's MedicAlert® plan with 24/7 Wandering Support) include links to "reverse 911" systems, which contact local police and hospitals to notify them that a person is missing. A Silver Alert system that notifies the public through their smartphones and highway billboards has been adopted by many states in an effort to locate lost people with dementia who may be traveling by car. The use and success are uncertain, but this program has increased many dementia families' awareness of the problem. High-tech solutions include tracking and GPS devices. Such devices must be routinely carried by the patient; however, many older people routinely carry cellular phones that have tracking systems and GPS built into the software. These programs allow linkage to other devices (e.g., the "find a smartphone" program) or allow for this information to be tracked on a computer. Other tools include GPS systems based in a small device attached to a key chain or embedded in the sole of a shoe. The big challenge is simply that the person must wear or carry the device at all times.

Medication errors

Errors in medication use are very common in people with dementia, and mistakes may go unrecognized for a long time. The potential risks of taking a medication too often include medication toxicity; taking medications too infrequently can lead to poor control of medical problems such as high blood pressure or diabetes. Poor medication adherence also makes it very difficult for the physician to organize a treatment plan because correct medication use is an important first step of most plans.

Medication compliance may be monitored by direct or indirect measures. Indirect measures are less precise but may provide helpful information about compliance; they start with determining whether prescriptions are being filled and refilled on a planned timeline. This allows for monitoring at a distance, but information on whether the medications are being taken as intended is limited. Unfortunately, people who are forgetful because of dementia often incorrectly report compliance.

Direct measures of medication compliance include observation and dispensing of medications by caregivers and offer much more reliable information. Several tools are also available to assist with medication compliance:

- Pill organizers (Figure 14.1) allow for tracking of whether medications were taken on a daily or weekly basis. Caregivers still need to fill the pill organizer with the prescribed medications on a weekly basis. Depending upon the layout of the pill organizer, pills can be separated into sections for the time of day (morning/evening or morning/noon/evening). At the end of the observation period (e.g., a

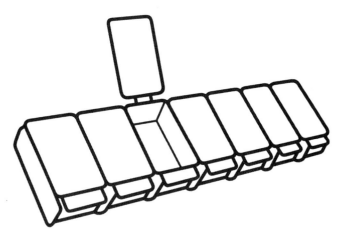

FIGURE 14.1 **A daily pill organizer.** The organizer has seven compartments, one for each day of the week. Some pill organizers have two or three compartments for each day to help with organizing medications taken more than once each day.

single day or week), the caregiver can determine whether the medications were taken (or at least are no longer in the pill organizer). More frequent observation (e.g., daily as opposed to weekly) can improve medication adherence. Some smartphone apps and calendar alerts provide automatic reminders that a dose of medication is due.

- Some pill bottles are "smart devices" that can record the timing and history of when a medication container was opened; the devices may also be able to communicate with a smartphone so caregivers can monitor medication adherence remotely. Some advanced pill organizers can hold a week or a month of medications and mechanically dispense each dose.
- Pharmacies may be able to prepare blister packs (Figure 14.2) of all medications to be dispensed in a given week.

Regardless of the approach taken, caregivers nearly always become increasingly involved with medication administration over the course of dementia.

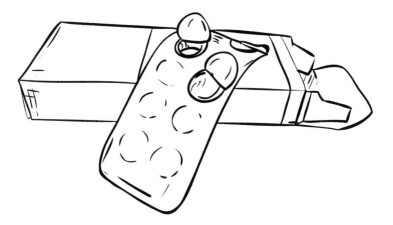

FIGURE 14.2 A blister pack for medications. A blister pack (or "multimed" pack) is a useful way that some pharmacies can prepare medications on a weekly basis. The medications are popped out of a small foil and plastic container.

Greta is 80 years old and has lived alone for much of her adult life ever since her husband died 25 years ago, when they were both in their 50s. She has remained active since then, including serving on her community board. At her annual physical exam, her primary care physician finds her blood pressure is elevated after years of good control. In response, her antihypertensive medication dose is increased. On a follow-up visit, her blood pressure is still elevated; in fact, it is now even higher than it was at the last two visits. A second antihypertensive medication is added. After discovering Greta is not taking her medications, her daughter takes on the responsibility of monitoring Greta's medications and starts attending all physician visits.

If medication use is not closely monitored, errors and poor outcomes become more likely. Proactive and preventive measures can identify the risk of medication noncompliance before catastrophic problems occur. Routine visits with a primary care physician can identify memory loss that may affect medication compliance through cognitive screening. Care partners or family members may also report memory loss and noncompliance.

Sometimes serious problems can follow long periods of unrecognized medication noncompliance. Failure to take medications as prescribed can lead to uncontrolled hypertension or diabetes, heart attack, stroke, and kidney failure. The sudden reintroduction of multiple medications that have been prescribed but not taken can also cause serious problems because of their effects and interactions. This can occur when a person with dementia has an involved caregiver for the first time. Unfortunately, examples like these happen all too often.

Fires and other household emergencies

The kitchen is one of the most welcoming and familiar places in a home. It is often the setting for socially rewarding and cognitively stimulating activities, including for people with dementia. The kitchen can also be one of the more dangerous places in the home for people with dementia, especially if it has not been adequately adapted or equipped for safety. Because of memory problems, people with dementia may leave a hot stove unattended or may not smell leaking natural gas or recognize it as dangerous. If a person with dementia must be left alone, removing the knobs on the stove can reduce the likelihood that they will light a fire unintentionally or leave the gas on. Household fires and other accidents, such as local flooding if a faucet is left running, need to be reported to the physician to ensure that more serious accidents do not happen. These events are important signals the doctor can use as the basis for referral to home care agencies and to meet the criteria of insurance companies, as these events demonstrate that there is an emerging risk at home that meets the threshold for home health services.

Family caregivers and health professionals should specifically ask how the person with dementia who still lives alone would respond to various hypothetical situations, including a kitchen fire. Using the household fire as an example, key questions to ask may include the following:

- What would you do if a grease fire broke out in the kitchen? (Acceptable answers: cover it, use a fire extinguisher, put baking soda on it; unacceptable answer: throw water on it.)
- What should you do if you see a fire in the home? (Acceptable answers: call 911, exit the home immediately; unacceptable answer: anything else, including calling a building supervisor or family member.)
- How can you prevent a fire from happening? (Acceptable answers: constant attention to meal preparation, ask someone else to cook, don't use the stove; unacceptable answer: anything else.)

Enhancing mobility and reducing the risk of falling

Falls can be catastrophic events in the course of dementia, especially if they are associated with hip or shoulder fracture or even brain injury.

Hospitalizations can be lengthy and complicated; even in the best-case scenario, full recovery may be limited.

The primary reasons people with dementia fall include accidental trips or slips; poor balance and the slow body movements seen in parkinsonism; falling out of bed due to rapid eye movement (REM) sleep behavior disorder, including dream enactment (Chapter 6); and fainting due to a drop in blood pressure (called **orthostatic hypotension**). Orthostatic hypotension occurs when a drop in blood pressure is not automatically corrected after a change in body position. These episodes of low blood pressure tend to occur when changing from a lying to a seated position or, more often, when changing from a seated to a standing position. Orthostatic hypotension may also occur just after passing urine or stool. Orthostatic hypotension often accompanies dementia with Lewy bodies and Parkinson's disease (Chapter 6). Treatments for orthostatic hypotension include making slow changes in body position (e.g., counting to 60 when sitting up from a lying position, standing up from a seated position, and, once standing, before starting to walk) and wearing compression stockings that squeeze the veins in the leg to prevent blood from pooling. Medication adjustments may be needed, including reducing the dose of medications being used to control high blood pressure or discontinuing them and introducing specific medications to increase blood pressure.

It is important to identify when someone is developing a risk for falling. Care partners can help by reporting any imbalance or near falls they have seen. A doctor's examination can identify imbalance and the stiffness and slowness of parkinsonism (Chapter 6). Red flags for fall risk at home include the following problems that may be noticed by care partners:

- Misjudging the position or height of chairs or beds, including episodes of narrowly missing or falling off of them
- Misjudging or tripping on stairs, steps, or uneven surfaces

- Cautiously holding on to furniture within the home (e.g., holding on to chairs, tables, and even walls, with each step) to maintain balance
- Symptoms of parkinsonism, including a slowed pace of walking relative to others, without problems in the joints (e.g., knee, ankle, or hip pain or instability)
- REM sleep behavior disorder, including dream enactment (acting out dreams at night with calling out and thrashing around)
- Orthostatic hypotension

Janet is a 68-year-old woman in the moderate stage of dementia with Lewy bodies. During a visit, her daughter observes that Janet often trips over the throw rugs in her home and holds on to the wall in the hallway when walking from her bathroom to the bedroom. Last week, she fell on her lawn while walking with her husband to the garden but did not break any bones when she landed on the soft soil. Her physician recommends using a four-wheel walker in her home to aid with stability. She is also referred to a physical therapist to devise a balance training exercise regimen that her husband can help her with at home. Gait and balance are tracked during future medical office visits.

The doctor may want to address any orthopedic problems (which often affect the knee) to improve balance or joint stability. Treatment options may include surgery or nonsurgical options such as bracing. When fall risk is identified, the doctor may attempt to minimize future risks by the following measures:

- Prescribing or recommending assistive devices for mobility, including a cane, conventional two-wheel walker or four-wheel rollator walker (typically with brakes and a seat; Figure 14.3).

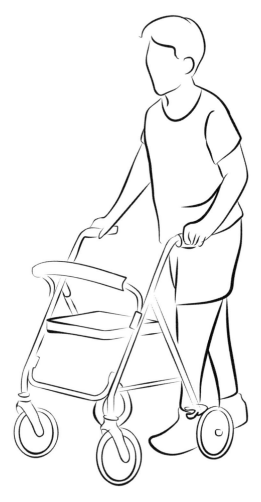

FIGURE 14.3 A four-wheel rollator walker. This style is a popular and sturdy option to help with mobility when walking in the community or at home. Key features include fully locking brakes and a seat. Some models can fold for portability.

A wheelchair may be necessary when away from home, such as at physician visits, but generally should be discouraged until necessary as it may decrease the amount of time spent standing or walking.

- Prescribing or recommending home safety devices, particularly in areas of high risk for falls. The area at highest risk for falls in the home is the bathroom. Installing grab bars on the walls of a shower and placing rubber floor mats in the tub will reduce the risk of falls. Shower/tub seats allow the patient to sit during a shower or bath. Some tub seat models allow the patient to slide sideways into the bathtub to eliminate the risk of falling while stepping over the high side of a bathtub. Figure 14.4 shows a bathtub set up with a shower seat and grab bars.
- Recommending ways to establish a safe environment in the bedroom to protect patients at risk for falling out of bed due to REM sleep behavior disorder. Suggestions may include moving

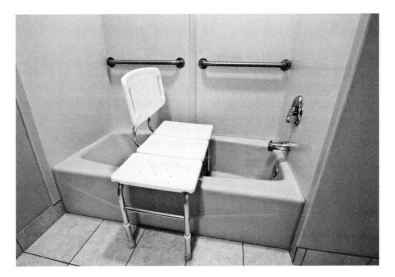

FIGURE 14.4 **A shower seat and grab bar.** This regular tub is set up with two key measures for bathroom safety. Two grab bars are installed on the wall to help with stability while standing and provide something to hold on to should the person feel off balance. Shower seats vary; the one pictured allows the person to sit down before entering the tub and then slide sideways. On some models, the seat itself slides sideways. The lower legs are lifted over the edge of the tub on both models.

the bed toward the wall, cushioning the side, and moving sharp objects (including furniture) away from the side of the bed. Installing bed rails may worsen the situation if the patient can climb over them. Bed alarms that sense changes in weight in the bed can alert others when the person arises unexpectedly.

- Referral to a physical therapist for gait assessment. With or without a **physiatrist** (rehabilitation doctor), a physical therapist can determine the most appropriate assistive device for walking (e.g., a cane or walker), establish an exercise regimen to be continued in the home, train a caregiver to perform exercises with the patient, and help identify risks at home.

- Referral for an in-home safety assessment. A patient's home may pose both obvious and unrecognized risks for falls, such as raised door thresholds and throw rugs. The slippery floors of the kitchen or bathroom and uneven surfaces, including stairs and thresholds between rooms, are places where falls are likely to occur. A home safety assessment will identify these risks and determine how they can be corrected.

Moving homes: when is the right time?

As needs change, moving the patient into a different home, adult community, or residential facility may begin to make sense. Moving may be motivated by the resources that are available in or around the home compared to those available elsewhere, safety needs (e.g., having everything on one floor instead of on different floors), or family considerations (e.g., moving closer to grandchildren). But moving at the wrong time can backfire, especially in the early to middle stages of dementia. At that point, the move itself may worsen the patient's confusion, agitation, and sundowning since familiar surroundings provide help with orientation in people with dementia. Unfortunately, it can be difficult to predict if a move will have a positive or negative outcome. It's wise to discuss this decision with the physician and family before moving.

Tools to enhance independence

Our technological world is increasingly dominated by personal hand-held computers. These devices include many tools that can be helpful, especially early in the course of dementia, such as calendar-based reminders and specialized apps with cognitive training programs. However, as dementia progresses, these devices often become increasingly difficult to operate or are forgotten altogether. Home safety alert pendants are very effective for people living independently without memory loss; they provide a personal safety net in case of falls and other medical emergencies. But when these devices are introduced after memory loss begins, a person with dementia may not use them due to confusion or may completely overlook them when they are needed.

As discussed earlier in this chapter, leaving a person with dementia alone can pose serious risks and is often associated with significant safety concerns. A system of personal and professional caregivers is most helpful but may not always be possible. Fortunately, new technology options, including in-home camera systems linked to the Internet, can enhance monitoring and safety. Advances in virtual monitoring include interconnected camera systems throughout the house that trigger alarms and deliver important real-time information. Such systems can be especially helpful during unwitnessed periods. These systems may extend the amount of time the person with dementia can continue to live independently at home yet provide immediate access to essential hands-on care. Of course, monitoring cannot eliminate risks, such as falls, but it nonetheless provides continuous surveillance for potential problems. These systems can be quite costly but may actually be cost-efficient relative to other options.

CHAPTER 15

Advance Care Planning

In this chapter, you will learn about:

- How to work with your friends, family, and doctor to plan for the future
- The differences between a health care proxy, will, living will, and durable power of attorney
- How to identify local resources to optimize strategies for advance care planning
- How different types of insurance function in supporting patient care
- Anticipating terminal decline and supporting the dying process
- How to remain focused on the primary goals of care throughout the course of dementia

Complex medical, financial, and legal issues can arise in each stage of dementia. Decisions about end-of-life and palliative care become increasingly important in late-stage dementia. An organized approach to learning how to navigate end-of-life decisions early on in dementia is helpful. These issues may arise when discussing other changes, such as stopping work and driving (Chapter 14). As is the case with most aspects of dementia care, planning ahead, ideally early in the disease course, with a patient-centered focus helps everyone involved to deliver the desired type of care. This chapter discusses how to effectively plan for the future through care transitions and the escalating care needs associated with dementia progression.

Advance care planning: an overview

Collectively, **advance care planning** refers to a range of important decisions about health care that should be considered by everyone, whether facing dementia or another illness or simply aging. Advance care planning involves considering goals of care and related decisions ahead of time and then letting others know about these preferences, including family members and doctors.

Engaging in discussions of advance care planning early on acknowledges and respects the wishes of the person facing dementia at a time when they can participate in the decision making and allows family members to come to a shared understanding. Moreover, having these conversations and agreeing on a plan early on allows important legal documents to be developed and available for use when needed. Some of these documents will guide care at later stages of the illness when persons are not able to make such decisions themselves. Understanding personal preferences is very helpful for a family member or other caregiver tasked with making difficult decisions.

Most people want to stay in their home for as long as possible, and this can be facilitated by making specific plans early on in dementia. However, staying in the home may not always be possible because of caregiver health issues, financial pressures, and competing obligations. The statistics are sobering: At least 50% of nursing home residents have dementia and more than one-third of dementia patients in advanced stages of disease will die in a nursing home. It's practical to focus on placing the patient's best interest, health, and long-standing preferences first. As the disease progresses, maintaining a high quality of care and safety may become more important than the earlier goal to stay in the home. Typically, these overarching goals are achievable and often support the well-being of both the patient and caregiver.

Formal legal matters

Several financial and legal considerations become increasingly important as dementia progresses as they are closely tied with important medical decisions, especially toward the end of life. The first step in advance care planning is understanding the role of several important legal documents. (None of the following should be considered legal advice; when in doubt, it's important to consult with an attorney.)

Relevant legal documents can be categorized into those related to health matters (e.g., **health care proxy**, **living will**) and those related to assets and management of personal property and financial matters (e.g., power of attorney, will). Advance care planning typically refers to legal documents related to how health care will be provided to someone in the future, but they are often created at the same time as other personal legal documents. For all of these documents, an attorney with experience in elder care issues should be consulted. If a personal attorney cannot be identified or is too costly, or if a caregiver is simply looking for a place to start, many local and national dementia advocacy groups provide support and counseling, including professional elder care attorneys (Appendix C).

Legal issues focused on personal assets

A full discussion of legal documents to secure personal wealth, as well as appropriate transfer of wealth and material possessions, is beyond the scope of this book. However, several terms are worth defining. **Wills** and **trusts** are the two principal tools to help dedicate funds during life to dementia care needs and allow for the funds remaining after death to be disbursed. Wills are typically created to direct a family member or **executor of an estate** to perform the actions spelled out in the document. Their responsibilities can range from making funeral arrangements to distributing wealth at the time of death. Living wills serve a very different purpose since they are not primarily focused on finances, and they are discussed later in this chapter. Trusts are legal documents establishing directors of financial management either during or after a person's lifetime and are typically referenced as a part of a will.

If a will was never written, each state determines how a decedent's remaining finances are handled and variably defaults to a mix of family and government-directed funds. If a person with advanced dementia lacks decision-making capacity and a responsible person to direct their care, most states have the means to appoint someone to manage their financial affairs. To ensure that money is spent in the best interest of the patient and in a manner that follows their wishes, early discussion and formal completion of legally recognized documents is important.

Legal issues focused on health

Several important legal documents can optimize the likelihood that a person's medical wishes will be followed and can diminish caregiver stress, especially if the documents are prepared before or shortly after dementia is diagnosed. These include a health care proxy and living will (also known as an advance directive or advance health care directive). Each document has a role in ensuring that the patient's preferences and needs are addressed in the context of medical decision making. These documents are often completed simultaneously and in a complementary manner, usually with the same people designated to make key decisions in each document. Completing these documents with involvement of the caregiver assures caregivers that their responsibilities and actions are clearly defined and can eliminate uncertainty and stress as people with dementia and their families face critical health problems.

Health care proxy

A **health care proxy**, sometimes called a medical power of attorney, is a document that legally designates a person as a **health care agent** appointed to make medical decisions for someone else when they cannot make decisions for themselves. Although technically the health care proxy is the document, the person who is a health care agent is often referred to as the health care proxy. Health care proxies can be temporary and can be revoked at any time. For example, temporary health care proxies are established for people undergoing elective surgery, even when good outcomes are expected. In contrast, health care proxies for older individuals tend to remain as initially designated (e.g., spouse). A backup or secondary health care proxy can also be designated at the time of completion of the form. This is important in case the primary health care proxy cannot be contacted, has become ill, or has died. Health care proxy forms are often completed at the time a patient enters a hospital, although a health care proxy created independent of a hospitalization can serve as a legal precedent as long as it has not been revoked or replaced. Although many health care proxy documents include a predetermined time window of validity, which may vary state to state, the most recent proxy is often honored, especially in times of medical emergencies.

The main purpose of the health care proxy document is so that a doctor or another health care provider knows who is designated to be responsible for a person's well-being. The designated health care proxy is typically expected to know the person well enough to act on their behalf even when questions and decisions posed have not previously been answered. Legally designated health care agents may consult with other individuals, but ultimately their decisions are followed for medical and legal purposes. In some states, if a person does not have the capacity to designate a health care agent legally through a health care proxy, then a **health care surrogate** may be identified to act as a health care agent. Persons designated through this process are the legal closest next of kin, a court-appointed guardian, or a close friend or other relative sufficiently familiar with the incapacitated person to be comfortable with and able to act on their known beliefs if a health care proxy is not available. A common example of a health care surrogate is when a spouse or domestic partner who has never been legally designated through a health care proxy is asked to make medical decisions following a person's sudden catastrophic illness. Barring a subsequently created health care proxy document, a health care surrogate document usually has the same legal resiliency as a health care proxy document and the individual serves the same purpose as a health care proxy, unless the surrogate defers decisions to the subsequent legal next of kin.

Power of attorney and durable power of attorney

A **power of attorney** is a document designating another person (the "attorney-in-fact") to be responsible for either some or all financial and legal actions if someone is briefly physically unavailable. A *durable* power of attorney gives the same responsibility but allows for this responsibility to be used when the designating person (e.g., a patient with cognitive impairment) is alive but becomes incapacitated or incompetent to make financial and legal decisions. The person designated as attorney-in-fact may also be a health care proxy, but these are usually established in separate legal documents that can be completed at the same time. Determination of an appropriate attorney-in-fact is a complex personal decision and requires designating someone who is considered trustworthy.

Decisional capacity is worth defining at this point, and people with dementia often retain it well into their illness. Decisional capacity, sometimes referred to as "competency," is typically determined by a medical professional and requires the physician to be convinced that the person is able to weigh and make medical decisions in the moment. Sometimes it takes a specialist to determine this (e.g., a psychiatrist or neurologist), but your primary doctor may be comfortable with making this determination. Decisional capacity can usually be determined in an interview in which the patient is told either real or hypothetical information and asked to repeat back what was told to them, make a decision, and explain why the decision was made. The point of the exercise is not to determine whether a patient makes a particular decision but rather to see if the patient makes a measured decision that could only be done using information that was provided in real time. As abilities in memory and verbal expression decline, so does decisional capacity.

Living wills and advance directives

Living wills (also known as **advance directives** or health care directives) are designed to direct a family member or a legally designated person to act on the expressed wishes of a person at a time when they become incapacitated. Any adult in any state of health may have an advance directive, and an advance directive may be changed over time depending on the person's wishes. It may also change in the context of certain diseases or if new treatments become available. Unlike a health care proxy, which designates an individual to act on a person's expressed desires whether or not specific health decisions had ever been discussed, advance directives provide a specific set of instructions and goals of care depending on one or more hypothetical health scenarios. In the context of dementia, specific points may relate to nutrition, hydration, and ventilator support, and these may depend on retained abilities and awareness by the person with dementia. It is difficult to think about many of these scenarios. Individuals with direct experience with end-of-life care (e.g., physicians or friends and family with personal experience) can be helpful in considering these complex issues and establishing a living will.

Code status: Do Not Resuscitate/Do Not Intubate

An important part of an advance directive is determining whether or not someone wants to be resuscitated or intubated when medically necessary. Resuscitation is the term used to describe steps to recover blood pressure and heart function through use of mechanical force (chest compressions), electrical means (shocking the heart), and medications (to treat abnormal heart rhythms or low blood pressure). Intubation involves placing a breathing tube into the mouth and throat when someone is unable to breathe on their own. A document or medical order determining that a patient is not to be resuscitated or intubated is called a Do Not Resuscitate/Do Not Intubate (DNR/DNI) determination, also known as "code status."

DNR/DNI can be assigned as temporary or permanent reflecting certain circumstances and can be determined by a health care proxy or as part of an advance directive. Many surgeries requiring general anesthesia and intubation temporarily revoke a DNR/DNI policy when intubation is a necessary part of the surgery. For the most part, DNR/DNI determinations are put into practice at a time when aggressive medical care would be considered futile or would only prolong suffering but may be applied during sudden unexpected illness. DNR/DNI determinations nearly always must be jointly signed. Since resuscitation and intubation are often used together, one cannot usually be just DNR or just DNI except in rare circumstances, such as when someone is already on permanent mechanical ventilation.

To help others know a patient's code status, a physician can complete a formal order that appears in medical record systems. This portable medical order has evolved under various names and is known as a **POLST** (now a term, previously an acronym for Physician's Orders for Life-Sustaining Treatment). The information contained in a POLST is, for the most part, the same information included in an advance directive. These are typically included in the medical record to provide guidance for critical decisions in the case of medical emergencies, including decisions for DNR/DNI.

Starting to think about and discuss advance care planning can be challenging. It is always best to start the conversation as early as possible, even before medical problems begin or worsen with age. Guidance on all these legal matters is part of several growing efforts, particularly the Five Wishes campaign. Created in 1998 by the nonprofit Aging with Dignity with support of the American Bar Association, end-of-life experts, and The Robert Wood Johnson Foundation, Five Wishes was designed to be "accessible, legal, and easy-to-understand with the goal of helping people discuss and document their wishes in a nonthreatening, life-affirming way." From a practical standpoint, Five Wishes is a tool to start conversations around matters of advance care planning with the goal of designating a health care proxy, creating an advance directive, and ensuring this information is shared with family members and doctors. This program also covers some subtle nonmedical issues about preferences in how care is delivered and received. Documentation through this program is legally recognized in 44 states and the District of Columbia, with recognition in all 50 as of early 2021 when used in association with state-level documents. A local dementia support organization or an elder care attorney may be able to provide additional assistance. Contact information for Five Wishes is available in Appendix C.

End-of-life care

Several important issues involving breathing, nutrition, and hydration become increasingly relevant as persons with dementia near the end of life.

Chewing, swallowing, and aspiration risk

Throughout the course of dementia, ensuring maintenance of good oral health habits is very important to optimize general health and nutrition. Establishing a routine for regular dental care as dementia progresses includes brushing teeth, flossing, and regular dentist visits. These steps help avoid or delay the need for dental procedures or surgical treatment of oral diseases that become increasingly difficult to accomplish later in dementia because of physical and cognitive changes. A number of assistive devices are available to support adequate brushing and flossing and to ensure dentures are maintained. Resources are listed in Appendix C.

In late-stage dementia, a range of bodily functions are affected, including chewing and swallowing. Choking on food and aspiration pneumonia are significant risks. Collectively, these changes in swallowing are termed **dysphagia**. Physicians will continually monitor patients with dementia for dysphagia. The history will generally reveal evidence of choking on food, and caregivers may recognize that some food consistencies are more problematic than others. It might be surprising to know that water and other thin liquids become especially difficult to swallow in later stages of dementia when swallowing is compromised. Liquids are hard to control and can slip right down into the lungs instead of the stomach. This is called aspiration, and an irritation and serious infection of the lungs called **aspiration pneumonia** can result.

Aside from obvious drooling or **dysarthria** (problems articulating speech), a neurologic examination for dysphagia may not be revealing. The problem shows itself during daily eating and drinking. The frequency and severity of choking should be monitored over time, and the doctor may suggest a **swallowing evaluation** when choking risk is suspected. Swallowing evaluations are performed by speech and language pathologists who are trained in identifying the cause of swallowing problems (and speech difficulties). Speech and language pathologists are able to recommend adaptive strategies, including how to change the consistency of food to reduce the risk of aspiration.

Supporting nutrition in late-stage dementia

When chewing and swallowing become difficult, a very challenging problem develops in how to continuously support nutrition and hydration. As dementia progresses, basic bodily functions, including chewing and swallowing, are affected, and nearly all people with dementia will need a change in the consistency of food. Swallowing problems may be short term (e.g., right after an acute illness such as pneumonia) or long term as dementia worsens. When swallowing is severely affected, food and water are supplied by **artificial nutrition and hydration** (sometimes called alternative nutrition and hydration). The primary options for providing artificial nutrition and hydration include intravenous fluids (fluids given by vein to support hydration) and tube feeding (for both nutrition and hydration). Liquid food may be given through either a feeding tube passed through the nose and down into the stomach (also called a nasogastric tube) or a tube that is surgically placed through the skin into the abdomen and into the stomach (also known as a gastrostomy tube) or the small intestine. For acutely ill hospitalized patients, nasal tube feedings are often used to maintain nutrition. Nasal tube feedings are generally safe when monitored closely and used appropriately for a relatively short period (e.g., days).

Long-term nutritional needs pose an increasing challenge, and liquid feedings are usually provided through a surgically implanted tube (Figure 15.1).

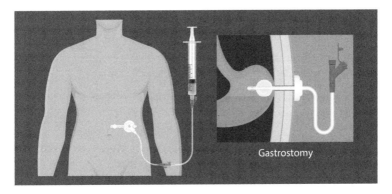

FIGURE 15.1 **A gastrostomy feeding tube.** Most often, a feeding tube is surgically placed through the skin of the upper abdomen with the tip sitting in the stomach. A plastic piece on the outside and a small balloon on the inside keep the tube secured. Bags of liquid food and water are given through a tube connected to a port at the end of the tube.

In rare circumstances, the gastrointestinal tract may not function properly, and nutrition will be given intravenously. Recent trends show that long-term tube feeding is being used less frequently in dementia as experience and research have shown the following:

- Tube feedings can prolong life but typically only during a period associated with poor quality of life for the patient and caregiver in the late stages of dementia.
- Attitudes have shifted because of changing personal preferences as expressed in advance directives, which are being used more often.
- Tube feeding does not change the risk of aspiration pneumonia; in people with severe swallowing problems, aspirating or inhaling saliva causes pneumonia just like accidentally inhaled food.
- Tube feedings are resource intensive, including the need for specialized caregivers or training and related equipment.
- Tube feedings can be complicated by unexpected breaks or rupture of the plastic tubing, infections around the site of insertion or in the abdomen, and unintentional removal of the tube, which may happen in a period of agitation. Therefore, tube feedings are a potential source of medical complications and even mortality.
- Maintaining the integrity of tube placement in the abdomen is difficult in an agitated person. In hospitalized patients, this leads to a cycle of using restraints and sedating medications to prevent a confused person from dislodging the feeding tube. These measures pose risk and limit mobility and participation in activities.

Family caregivers need the time to speak with other family members and their physicians to make the best decisions about tube feeding and other issues at the end of life. Discussions about nutrition are highly individualized, with some families expressing discomfort at the thought of withholding nutrition. Deciding either to provide or not provide tube feedings is acceptable.

Sometimes family members may consider failing to provide food or water to be the same as "no care." To alleviate the potential caregiver distress when no food or water is being given, an alternative is **comfort feeding**. In comfort feeding, small quantities of food are hand fed to the patient as long as obvious choking does not follow. Comfort feeding does not generally hasten death or prolong life. Providing some nutrition through comfort feeding, even if inadequate relative to a person's nutritional needs, can be helpful in alleviating caregiver and family distress.

No matter which approach is taken, it is best to make these decisions early, before they are urgent. Once a person with dementia is no longer able to sustain sufficient intake of liquids, dehydration develops and death usually follows in a matter of days.

Supporting ventilation in late-stage dementia

Mechanical ventilation is an artificial means to support breathing using a device that either inflates the lungs or assists with each breath. Breathing support is delivered either through a device placed over the nose and mouth or through a tube placed in the **trachea** (the windpipe) by a surgical procedure. With the exception of amyotrophic lateral sclerosis associated with frontotemporal dementia (Chapter 7) or devastating stroke (Chapter 8), breathing support is rarely necessary in most forms of dementia. Breathing problems that would require ventilator support nearly always begin long after swallowing problems. In frontotemporal dementia with amyotrophic lateral sclerosis, noninvasive mechanical ventilation is a treatment option. This involves a mask that is placed over the mouth and nose that helps keep the lungs inflated well with each breath. This can sustain life, and most patients and families find that it sustains a meaningful quality of life, if even for a brief period. Amyotrophic lateral sclerosis care is covered in depth in *Navigating Life with Amyotrophic Lateral Sclerosis* by Mark B. Bromberg, MD, PhD, FAAN, and Diane Banks Bromberg, JD (Oxford University Press, 2017).

Hospice and dying

With few exceptions, the course of dementia involves progressive cognitive, behavioral, and physical decline. Even when patients are significantly affected by dementia with limited language production and mobility, the gradual decline can continue for years. **Hospice** is a component of palliative care (See Chapter 10) and offers more intensive multimodal and interdisciplinary approaches to care focused on alleviating or ameliorating suffering in the process of dying. Hospice is generally available for patients with any condition once the patient's life expectancy is estimated to be 6 months or less. Pain and discomfort are the targets of medical care in hospice settings. Disease-specific treatments, such as chemotherapy for cancer, can continue to be used in hospice if the treatment alleviates suffering such as pain from a tumor.

Hospice typically occurs in dedicated centers that aim to create a welcoming and supportive environment for family members and other care partners, often allowing and encouraging around-the-clock visits, or at home through home hospice programs which include visits by health professionals who work with personal and professional caregivers to deliver care. Hospice can also be delivered through teams offering hospice care in hospitals or nursing homes. Hospice professionals are especially skilled at providing support to family and other caregivers and grief counseling to help cope with the dying process and loss.

Because of the challenges of determining life expectancy in dementia until very late stages, most insurance providers require strict criteria to be met to qualify for hospice, as determined by the **Functional Assessment Staging Tool** (FAST). Patients with dementia qualify for hospice once their spontaneous speech output is down to a few words every day, they are unable to stand, and they have experienced a recent illness associated with immobility, such as a decubitus ulcer (bedsore), urinary tract infection, aspiration pneumonia, blood clot, or persistent fever of unknown source. These are generally the causes of death for dementia patients, although an array of related or unrelated neurologic disorders (e.g., seizures and stroke) and unrelated non-neurologic disorders (e.g., heart disease and cancer) may emerge in patients with dementia, especially in patients with a long course.

Admission to a hospice center or receiving hospice services at home involves certain agreements to establish a shared understanding of the goals of care. Often, hospice involves "capping" of care. Capping is the decision not to treat a recurring problem or new problem or to treat a recurring problem less aggressively the next time. For example, if a feeding tube is unintentionally removed, an agreement may include that the patient will not return to the hospital for it to be replaced. In hospice, a central theme is to look a few steps ahead to help inform the goals of care. If a new medical diagnosis arises (e.g., acute stroke), issues driving care decisions can include the invasiveness of diagnostic tests required (e.g., CT scan), steps necessary to get the test (e.g., hospitalization), and the type of intervention (e.g., ranging from new medications requiring blood monitoring to even surgery). Some decisions may have no impact on quality of life, whereas others may worsen quality of life. In most cases, the stress involved with certain paths of treatment or potential complications following hospitalization are taken into consideration.

Physician-assisted dying

Physician-assisted dying (or medical aid in dying) is an important topic in dementia with complex medicolegal concerns. At present, legal statutes have been considered on a state-by-state basis and in several countries outside the United States. Physician-assisted dying involves a voluntary request by a person to receive a prescription medication from a physician to hasten death in a peaceful and humane manner. Depending on where the request occurs and when in the course of disease it occurs, it may or may not be legally acceptable. For physician-assisted dying to be considered, patients must participate voluntarily on their own behalf and meet eligibility at the time of a request, including the retained ability to enact a voluntary decision. The very nature of the cognitive impairment in late-stage dementia impacts decision making, making physician-assisted dying in dementia ethically challenging and exceptionally rare.

Insurance

The cost of care for dementia in the United States, particularly in the later stages, is very high. The daily cost to stay in a nursing home is about as much as staying in a midrange hotel room. It is not uncommon for long-term residential care programs to cost upward of $100,000 per year, depending on the services needed. Some people with advanced dementia may require high-level expensive care for years (Chapter 3). Medical or health insurance often determines what medical and supportive services may be made possible or affordable to patients. In the United States, some government-supported insurance programs offer more services (e.g., Medicaid) than others. Typically, patients must pay to use services if they have financial means to pay for such services. Medicare and some private health insurance companies generally do not cover supportive services. Any potential assets, including real estate, are usually counted against someone's financial bottom line and, until liquidated, can make receiving outside support (such as through Medicaid) next to impossible.

Although much of care is determined by costs supported by medical insurance, long-term care insurance policies can help defray the costs of care. **Long-term care insurance policies** generally need to be purchased by adults before (and often well before) the seventh decade of life. Having a preexisting condition or certain genetic risks may increase the insurance premium or deem a person uninsurable. In the United States, genetic discrimination protections generally only apply to health insurance and not to long-term care insurance programs. Long-term care insurance can be a valuable investment but often needs to be purchased at a time in life when people have many other financial obligations related to growing families. Typically, long-term care insurance allows for a fixed period of time of financial support related to late-life care. The amount of compensation per day and the total period of time covered (the number of years the policy can be used) vary and often impact the price of the policy. Many long-term care insurance policies cover most, if not all, of the care needs at the end stage of disease. Some are time limited, perhaps covering up to 5 years of time. Because of the time-dependent nature of policies, many families opt to not use the policies until moderate to late-stage disease has been identified.

As detailed earlier, the prognosis of dementia is very hard to predict, and an argument can be made for beginning to use long-term care insurance policies earlier in the disease. Doing so before financial burdens of dementia significantly increase, and while a person with dementia still has some degree of independence, may support a more active life for caregivers and provide greater personal reward. Early use of a long-term care policy may enable around-the-clock caregiver assistance in the home and respite care for family members. Recognizing the significant financial burden of informal caregiving (e.g., family members missing work) and the special connections family members have, some long-term care policies will pay for family members to serve as professional caregivers, defraying some of the income lost through informal caregiving.

Epilogue

Whether you read this book as a caregiver or are facing dementia yourself, by the time you have explored it to better understand how life will change, life will likely have already changed. No two journeys through the course of dementia are alike. No two people experience dementia for the same amount of time, have the same types of symptoms, or experience symptoms to the same degree. What is certain is that life does change meaningfully for each individual over the course of this illness.

In both the realms of research and clinical care, scientists and physicians continue to work toward a time when better treatments are available that will make a meaningful difference in slowing decline in Alzheimer's disease and other dementias. However, many aspects of this book will likely nevertheless remain relevant for some time to come.

Until dementia is eliminated, it is important to try to find as much joy in the smallest moments as often as possible. Think about how to make the best of ordinary moments despite the problems created by cognitive impairment and behavioral changes. Find enjoyable activities that do not require a forgetful person to remember things from moments ago. For people with language impairment, these could be outlets for nonverbal expression and engagement. In late-stage dementia, having a set plan for daily and weekly activities can help make routine care and brief excursions outside the home more manageable.

No matter the stage of disease or type of impairments, people with dementia can derive some joy in life, often at unexpected times. Caregivers need to find joy too. Art, music, dance, and planned activities can improve the sense of well-being for all and may help address apathy and anger, with very little risk involved.

With memory and emotional problems sometimes changing moment to moment, the challenges and problems faced in the moment (the "now") also have to be addressed. Being strong and prepared for problems will help in hard times. Setting a positive tone, providing simple explanations, and redirecting thoughts or changing the subject can be very effective ways to diffuse behavioral problems. Be supportive when problems with communication arise rather than pointing them out and causing unnecessary stress. Fundamentally, these challenges have no easy answers or solutions. It requires on-your-feet thinking, creativity, and flexibility in ever-changing scenarios.

Certainly, suffering and challenges in life are not unique to dementia, and this is not the first book to give some guidance and wisdom to major existential challenges in life. In his short story "The Three Questions," first published in 1885, Leo Tolstoy told of a king who wanted to succeed at everything he might undertake. After rejecting answers he received from many learned subjects, including counselors, priests, and doctors, he settled on asking a certain wise hermit: "How can I learn to do the right thing at the right time? Who are the people I most need, and to whom should I, therefore, pay more attention than to the rest? And, what affairs are the most important, and need my first attention?" The answers are, of course, complex and unique to each life journey, whether or not dementia is involved. But after the king unexpectedly helped a hermit heal an injured stranger who had been planning to kill him, Tolstoy's wise hermit eventually answered, encouraging the king to live in the moment: "Remember then: there is only one time that is important—Now! It is the most important time because it is the only time when we have any power. The most necessary man is he with whom you are, for no man knows whether he will ever have dealings with anyone else: and the most important affair is, to do him good, because for that purpose alone was man sent into this life!"

So now is the time for us all to act—to have a specific diagnosis made, to begin treatment, to share what you have learned in this book, to be a part of an evolving new era of disease-modifying therapies in dementia, to plan for the future, and to find ways to enjoy the moments immediately ahead. I hope you have found this handbook useful to discover ways to help the person you are with, doing some good in their life, despite dementia itself. May a next edition of this book provide more hope and share news of better treatments.

APPENDIX A

Nuclear Medicine Imaging

Understanding how nuclear medicine imaging techniques work starts by understanding how basic x-rays and related studies function. Standard x-rays and CT scans involve the projection of x-rays from a machine into the patient to see how energy is absorbed and transmitted through the body. The captured image can show the structure of the body part but not how it is functioning. **Nuclear medicine** techniques allow a window into seeing how parts of the body are working. Nuclear medicine studies involve giving the patient a **radiolabeled** or "tagged" substance, usually via an intravenous catheter (IV) in an arm, which then circulates throughout the body. In the case of brain imaging, these substances settle into the brain, emit a signal from certain regions, and highlight the function (or dysfunction) of part of the brain or a related specific ongoing process. Current nuclear medicine techniques do not provide a high-resolution image as can be seen on MRIs and instead show relative differences of signal over larger areas of the brain. In the field of nuclear medicine for dementia, the techniques can be broadly split into those identifying **brain metabolism** and those identifying brain pathologic processes.

Nuclear medicine studies demonstrating brain metabolism include **positron emission tomography** (PET) tagged with a **glucose** or sugar molecule (FDG-PET) and **single-photon emission computed tomography** (SPECT), which measures brain perfusion. The current leading hypothesis for why these tests help us in making a diagnosis is that the areas of the brain most strongly associated with neuropathologic evidence of dementia are those in which the brain cells (neurons) are most dysfunctional. Areas with dysfunctional neurons are less metabolically demanding and therefore require less glucose (sugar), which is thus taken up less in these areas. The brain may also have a relatively lower demand for oxygenated blood in these regions. A brain FDG-PET scan demonstrates relative areas of glucose metabolism, whereas brain SPECT demonstrates relative areas of brain perfusion. Patterns of low metabolism or low perfusion are generally similar across these techniques, and the techniques are thus used somewhat interchangeably.

From a practical standpoint, most insurance companies in the United States will not pay for FDG-PET unless the patient is at least 65 years old and certain specific forms of dementia are being considered. The value of these tests in distinguishing uncommon causes of dementia is less certain. An important limitation of both brain FDG-PET and brain SPECT is related to how intact the brain regions of interest are. That is, an area of the brain that is relatively small, shrunken, or atrophied would be expected to have low signal not because of low metabolism or perfusion but because there is less brain volume in that area in the first place. PET or SPECT imaging showing lower signal in areas with a sufficiently large regional brain volume can be more reliable in judging what changes may be under way.

Although patterns of low metabolism or low perfusion shown on FDG-PET and SPECT can be helpful in refining the diagnosis of dementia, they cannot definitively show what is causing the changes. Nonetheless, the patterns can be very instructive if they are clearly normal or match a typical or common pattern of dementia, such as AD.

Newer to the biomarker field is PET imaging, which instead reflects the pathologic changes of dementia. At present, several FDA-approved substances can be used in PET imaging to diagnose amyloid- and tau-related changes in the brain. A negative or normal amyloid-PET scan strongly argues against the presence of AD or a related disorder such as cerebral amyloid angiopathy. But a negative amyloid scan cannot determine the presence or absence of other related dementias, such as dementia with Lewy bodies, frontotemporal dementia, and others. The tau-PET scans available are specific to diagnosing AD, at least its later stages. Additional PET techniques reflecting other pathologic brain protein changes (such as α-synuclein) are of interest and in various phases of development. Until recently amyloid-PET and tau-PET were not paid for by insurance companies, given that they had no bearing on treatment. However, amyloid-PET may soon be supported given the recent availability of disease-modifying therapies in AD, and the need to confirm a biologically based diagnosis before starting treatment.

APPENDIX B

The Lumbar Puncture

The process by which cerebrospinal fluid (CSF) is obtained is called a lumbar puncture or spinal tap. Many people react to the thought of getting a lumbar puncture with fear or immediate dismissal. This reaction is probably unwarranted and may principally relate to lack of familiarity. For most patients, lumbar punctures are performed safely in a neurologist's office.

The main steps of a lumbar puncture are nearly identical to those performed during spinal anesthesia given in the course of childbirth. The procedure begins with the patient either seated or lying on one side. The doctor will try to get the patient into a position to bend the lower back as much as possible, as shown in the figure B.1. Several parts of the hip bones and lower backbone serve as landmarks to guide the doctor in finding the right place to insert the needle. After making sure the location is correct, the area will be carefully cleaned and special paper will cover the area to make sure the skin stays sterile. Once the skin is cleaned and a sterile field has been created, the physician may again palpate, or feel, the hips and spine to make sure that the patient remains aligned and positioned appropriately.

At this point, a numbing medication is injected into the skin and later into the deep tissues in the back using a small needle. Typically, a local anesthetic medication called **lidocaine** is used; this is the same medication used in most dental procedures or in dermatologist offices

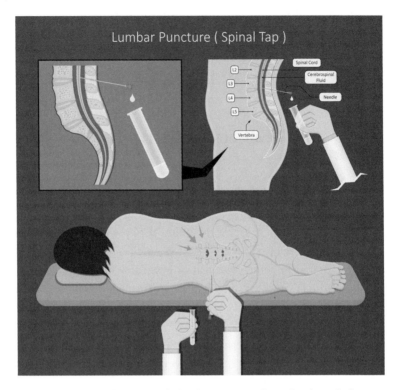

FIGURE B.1 **Performance of a lumbar puncture (spinal tap).** With the patient in either a seated or lying position, a needle is inserted through the lower back and into the spinal canal. The CSF drips out slowly and is collected and analyzed. Here, the patient is shown lying on the left side.

for minor procedures, including biopsy. After waiting a few moments to ensure the anesthetic has taken effect, the spinal needle is placed into the lower back. This needle is the same size (or sometimes smaller in diameter) than the needles used in drawing blood but is longer as it needs to reach the area of fluid in the spinal canal. Based on the manner of positioning just described, the neurologist will target the level of the spinal canal below which the spinal cord has ended, eliminating the risk of the needle injuring the spinal cord. Despite careful positioning, the neurologist may need to insert the needle several times before CSF begins flowing. Once the needle is correctly positioned, it is simply a matter of waiting for the CSF to drip out of the needle. In most cases, the process of setting up the lumbar puncture and cleaning up afterward takes longer than the process of actually inserting the needle and collecting the fluid, and start to finish is usually less than an hour. Once the lumbar puncture is complete, the early results will usually become available within days, although some of the test results may take several weeks to return.

Sometimes a lumbar puncture is not so easy. For patients with lower-back arthritis or a history of back surgery, a lumbar puncture may need to be done under a radiologist's guidance, using x-ray to ensure appropriate positioning during the procedure. The machines required for x-ray assessment are similar to those used in the angiographic, or blood vessel, imaging that is required for coronary or heart vessel angiography. In that case, patients are usually referred to a hospital or outpatient radiologic facility capable of doing these and related procedures.

The main reason why a lumbar puncture cannot be done is that the patient is taking medications that cause the blood to clot more slowly (**anticoagulation** medications), such as those taken for atrial fibrillation, artificial heart valves, or other reasons. In some circumstances, medications can be adjusted to allow a lumbar puncture to be performed, but this usually requires a coordinated effort to switch the patient from oral to injectable anticoagulation medications. Relevant blood levels will need to be monitored to ensure that anticoagulation remains in place except for a few hours around the time of the lumbar puncture.

Most of the time, lumbar punctures are very safe. The most common side effect is a headache afterward, but even this occurs in a small number of patients and often goes away shortly after the test is over. The brain and related structures have about 120 to 150 milliliters (about 12 tablespoons) of CSF, and most lumbar punctures require removing about 10 to 20 milliliters of fluid (around 1 tablespoon).

The adult brain creates about 15 milliliters of CSF each hour. So by the time the patient leaves the physician's office after a lumbar puncture, the CSF volume that was removed will mostly be replaced. Nonetheless, about 1 in 6 to 10 people will experience a headache after the lumbar puncture that is worsened when they sit or stand up. Innovations in needle-tip design have substantially decreased the risk of these headaches. Although for many years routine practice was to advise a patient to remain lying flat after a lumbar puncture, it is probably more important to avoid heavy lifting or stooping for 1 to 2 days.

Sometimes people feel some brief tingling in the legs or feet during a lumbar puncture. Insertion of the needle itself is not painful, given that the skin and structures just beneath it that have greater pain perception than the deeper structures are premedicated with a local anesthetic, as described earlier. Those structures may instead produce a perception of pressure where the needle is inserted. However, a minor amount of pain may be perceived as the spinal needle is advanced into deeper structures beyond the reach of the anesthetizing needle. This pain is usually limited and not debilitating. Because of the local injury related to introducing the spinal needle into the lower back, there may be some bruising and soreness at the site of the lumbar puncture for 1 to 2 days after the procedure.

APPENDIX C

Resources

While the Internet can be a wonderful and immediately accessible resource for information, it also comes with the risk of misinformation, and this is especially true of medical information. The resources included in this appendix include trusted sites that primarily provide information that is based on facts and tested data, particularly those provided by the National Institutes of Health. Also included in this appendix is a listing of nonprofit organizations engaged in the support of patients with specific types of dementia and their caregivers. Additionally, through each of these organizations, there are often links to local chapters that may provide additional local information and resources about the communities they serve. By no means is this a comprehensive list, but it includes resources that are typically known to be reliable and useful.

General Resources

Dementia, General

National Institutes of Health: ninds.nih.gov/Disorders/All-Disorders/Dementia-Information-Page
Alzheimers.gov

This is the United States federal government's portal to information and resources on Alzheimer's disease and related dementias, managed by the National Institute on Aging: https://www.alzheimers.gov/

World Health Organization: who.int/news-room/fact-sheets/detail/dementia

Caregiving in Dementia

National Institutes of Health: nia.nih.gov/health/alzheimers/caregiving

National Institutes of Health: nidcr.nih.gov/health-info/for-older-adults

National Institute on Aging: nia.nih.gov/health/taking-care-your-teeth-and-mouth

Well Spouse, 63 West Main St., Ste. H, Freehold, NJ 07728; Phone: 800-838-0879; wellspouse.org

Respite Care Resources

Access to Respite Care and Help (ARCH); includes respite care locator: archrespite.org/

Resources (Alphabetical by Disease)

Alzheimer's Disease

National Institutes of Health: https://www.nia.nih.gov/alzheimers/publication/alzheimers-disease-fact-sheet

National Institute on Aging and the National Plan to Address Alzheimer's Disease: nia.nih.gov/about/nia-and-national-plan-address-alzheimers-disease

National Institute on Aging's webpage on Alzheimer's Disease
Research Centers: nia.nih.gov/research/adc
Support organizations
   Alzheimer's Association, National Office, 225 N. Michigan
      Ave., Fl. 17, Chicago, IL 60601
   Phone: 800-272-3900; alz.org
   Alzheimer's Disease International, 57A Great Suffolk St.,
      London, SE1 0BB UK
   Phone: +44 20 79810880; alzint.org
   Alzheimer's Foundation of America, 322 Eighth Ave, 16th Fl.,
      New York, NY 10001
   Phone: 866-232-8484; alzfdn.org

CADASIL

National Institutes of Health: ninds.nih.gov/Disorders/All-
Disorders/CADASIL-Information-Page
Cure CADASIL, 10 Schalks Crossing Rd., Ste. 501A-133,
Plainsboro, NJ 08536; curecadasil.org

Creutzfeldt–Jakob Disease

National Institutes of Health: ninds.nih.gov/Disorders/All-
Disorders/Creutzfeldt-Jakob-Disease-Information-Page
Support organization
   Creutzfeldt-Jakob Disease Foundation, Inc., 3634 W. Market
      St., Akron, OH 44333
   HelpLine: 800-659-1991; cjdfoundation.org

Depression

National Institutes of Health: nimh.nih.gov/health/topics/
depression/index.shtml

Disorders of Metabolism

National Institutes of Health: genome.gov/Genetic-Disorders/
Inborn-Errors-of-Metabolism

Epilepsy

National Institutes of Health: ninds.nih.gov/Disorders/All-
Disorders/Epilepsy-Information-Page
Support organizations
    American Epilepsy Society, 135 S. LaSalle St., Ste. 2850,
       Chicago, IL 60603
    Phone: 312-883-3800; aesnet.org
    International League Against Epilepsy, 2221 Justin Rd., Ste.
       119-352, Flower Mound, TX 75028
    Phone: 860-586-7547; ilae.org

Frontotemporal Dementia

National Institutes of Health: ninds.nih.gov/Disorders/All-
Disorders/Frontotemporal-Dementia-Information-Page
Support organization
    Association for Frontotemporal Degeneration, 2700 Horizon
       Dr., Ste. 120, King of Prussia, PA 19406
    HelpLine: 866-507-7222; theaftd.org

Huntington's Disease

National Institutes of Health: ninds.nih.gov/Disorders/All-
Disorders/huntingtons-Disease-Information-Page
Support organization
    Huntington's Disease Society of America, 505 Eighth Ave.,
       Ste. 902, New York, NY 10018
    Helpline: 800-345-HDSA (4372); National Office: 212-242-1968
    Email: HDSAinfo@HDSA.org; hdsa.org

Leukodystrophies

National Institutes of Health: rarediseases.info.nih.gov/diseases/
6895/leukodystrophy
Support organization
    United Leukodystrophy Foundation, 224 N. Second St., Ste.
      2,DeKalb, IL 60115
      Phone: 800-728-5483; 815-748-3211; ulf.org

Lewy Body Disease

National Institutes of Health: nia.nih.gov/alzheimers/
publication/lewy-body-dementia/introduction
Support organization
    Lewy Body Dementia Association, 912 Killian Hill Rd. SW,
      Lilburn, GA 30047
      Phone: 800-539-9767; http://lbda.org

Multiple Sclerosis

National Institutes of Health: ninds.nih.gov/Disorders/All-
Disorders/Multiple-Sclerosis-Information-Page
Support organization
    National Multiple Sclerosis Society, P.O Box 4527, New York,
      NY 10163
      Phone: 800-344-4867; nationalmssociety.org/

Normal Pressure Hydrocephalus

National Institutes of Health: ninds.nih.gov/Disorders/All-
Disorders/Normal-Pressure-Hydrocephalus-Information-Page
Support organization
    Hydrocephalus Association, 4340 East West Highway, Suite
      905, Bethesda, MD 20814-4447

Phone: 301-202-3811/888-598-3789; hydroassoc.org/
normal-pressure-hydrocephalus/

Progressive Supranuclear Palsy

National Institutes of Health: ninds.nih.gov/Disorders/All-
Disorders/Progressive-Supranuclear-Palsy-Information-Page
Support organization
    Cure PSP, 1216 Broadway, 2nd Floor, New York, NY 10001
    Phone: 800-457-4777/347-294-2873 (CURE); 844-287-3777
    (Canada); psp.org

Schizophrenia

National Institutes of Health: nimh.nih.gov/health/topics/
schizophrenia/index.shtml

Suicide Prevention

National Institutes of Health: nimh.nih.gov/health/topics/
suicide-prevention/index.shtml
National Suicide Prevention Lifeline: 1-800-273-TALK (8255);
suicidepreventionlifeline.org/

Traumatic Brain Injury

National Institutes of Health: ninds.nih.gov/Disorders/All-
Disorders/Traumatic-Brain-Injury-Information-Page
Support organization
    Brain Injury Association of America, 3057 Nutley St #805,
    Fairfax, VA 22031
    Phone: 703-761-0750; biausa.org; National Brain Injury
    Information Center: 1-800-444-6443

Vascular Cognitive Impairment

National Institutes of Health:
   ninds.nih.gov/Disorders/Clinical-Trials/
      Post-stroke-Cognitive-Impairment-and-Dementia
   ninds.nih.gov/disorders/all-disorders/
      stroke-information-page
Support organization
   American Stroke Association (a division of the American
   Heart Association), National Center, 7272 Greenville Ave.,
   Dallas, TX 75231
   Phone: 800-AHA-USA-1 (800-242-8721); strokeassociation.
      org/

Dementia Research Resources

The following are listings of all ongoing and past registered clinical
trials, including those focused on specific dementia diseases that are
ongoing in specific geographic areas:

   Europe: European Clinical Trials Database (EudraCT), managed
      by the European Medicines Agency: eudract.ema.europa.eu/
   United States: Clinical trials managed by the U.S. National
      Library of Medicine. This covers all U.S. and many
      international registered clinical trials: clinicaltrials.gov

The Alzheimer's Association's Trial Match Program can be
accessed at trialmatch.alz.org/find-clinical-trials#createaccount.
   Up-to-date information about the status of major Alzheimer's research can be found at the Alzheimer's Research Forum (alzforum.
org).
   The journal *Alzheimer's & Dementia* annually publishes a summary called the 'Alzheimer's disease drug development pipeline' and

can be found by searching for that title through the National Library of Medicine. https://www.ncbi.nlm.nih.gov/pmc/

Advance Care Planning

Elder Care Legal Assistance

National Academy of Elder Law Attorneys; Phone: 703-942-5711; naela.org

Physician's Orders for Life-Sustaining Treatment

National POLST, 208 I Street NE, Washington DC 20002; Phone: 202-780-8352; Polst.org

Advance Directives

Five Wishes (Aging with Dignity), P.O. Box 1661, Tallahassee, FL 32302-1661; Office Location: 3050 Highland Oaks Terrace, Ste. 2, Tallahassee, FL 32301-3841; fivewishes.org

Clinical Trials and Other Research Study Opportunities

Everything that we know about dementia comes from the efforts of researchers and dedicated clinical trial participants. Without this ongoing commitment to research, our knowledge would remain stalled where it is now, with few effective therapies for most forms of dementia. Participating in research is an option that all people affected by dementia should be aware of. Having more persons with dementia become involved in research is expected to more rapidly advance the discovery of dementia causes and treatments. All trials, even "failed" ones, have led to new discoveries and even challenged the fundamental beliefs of how diseases like Alzheimer's affect the brain. Participating in research is a personal decision that should be informed by several important considerations.

Types of research studies

Research studies are broadly categorized as being observational or interventional.

Observational studies typically follow patients over time or perform assessments, including history and physical examination, neuropsychological studies, imaging, or fluid-based studies (drawing blood or obtaining cerebrospinal fluid). Other studies offer opportunities for a post-mortem brain examination, or brain autopsy, the ultimate gift to research. Each additional brain autopsy leads to a better understanding of dementia. All of these study designs have offered great insight into understanding the **pathophysiology**, or cause, of disease, its prognosis, and its natural history; in some cases, they offer opportunities for refining the diagnosis and impacting care.

In **interventional studies**, also known as treatment studies, a medication, treatment, or "intervention" is given to someone with dementia and the results are compared with those from others who do not get the medication to find out if the treatment made a difference.

Dementia research has seen several shifts over the past decade and has benefited from a broader base of research awareness, as researchers are now studying a broader range of types of dementias and those with earlier symptoms. Historically, most research in dementia has focused on Alzheimer's disease. Alzheimer's-focused studies continue to include both observational and interventional studies; however, research is trending away from observational studies to those more focused on treatment in hopes of finding effective disease-modifying therapies. More recently, the less common dementias have become part of major research efforts: Some of the same study designs that had been used previously in Alzheimer's disease are now being used in frontotemporal dementia and dementia with Lewy bodies. At present, observational studies are more common than interventional studies in non-Alzheimer's dementias.

In recent years, treatment studies have become more focused on individuals who have early-stage dementia or are even presymptomatic rather than those with later-stage illness. By the time that the later stages of dementia develop, the brain has undergone major changes that seem to be irreversible. Treatments used earlier in dementia may help slow decline at a time when the brain still has a chance to respond in an obvious meaningful way. However, new symptom-based treatments are being offered for all stages of disease, so options for treatment trials are still available no matter the stage of dementia.

Is research right for me?

Patients and families may have several motivating reasons for participating in research. However, before participating in research, they should consider the following:

- Patients and families who get involved in research should do so with the understanding that it is for the greater good, to aid in better understanding of the disease, and not with the expectation of deriving direct personal benefit. Dedicated individuals are needed to move the field forward and, it is hoped, to find more effective treatments.
- To date, no medication has proven beneficial as a disease-modifying therapy.
- Sometimes it is learned that trial medications are not safe, even if earlier smaller studies suggested they were safe.
- For most treatment trials, half of the enrolled participants do not receive the drug being tested but instead receive a **placebo** (or no active treatment) and do not find out until the end of the study.
- Participation in research requires a personal commitment to begin and follow through with all research steps, which may involve a significant time commitment by both the person with dementia and a study partner (often the primary caregiver).
- Many, but not all, current dementia studies require additional imaging, including MRI and PET, bloodwork, and even cerebrospinal fluid analysis.
- Every study has strict inclusion and exclusion criteria (including age, diagnosis, medical history, medications, and other criteria).
- Most studies take place through research centers, but not all research centers offer the same studies or all current studies.
- All research is supervised and organized to ensure that participants' safety and autonomy remain central in any new investigational drug test.

- People participating in research studies are not asked to pay to participate. Most participants in research are modestly compensated for their time.
- The window of opportunity for enrollment into a specific study can be quite short, sometimes only weeks to months long.
- One particular phase of trial may be of greater interest. **Phase 2 studies** focus on the safety of a treatment but may provide early signals of efficacy, whereas treatments in **phase 3 studies** have already demonstrated some safety and the focus is on efficacy.

If research is a good fit after considering these points, the first step in enrolling is to complete the research center's determination of study eligibility (including age, diagnosis, medical history, and medications, among other criteria).

GLOSSARY

Advance care planning: broadly refers to all matters of planning for the future but is typically used when making plans for the future regarding health matters, including designating a health care proxy, creating a living will, and creating a plan to communicate this information to family, friends, and physicians

Advance directive: see *living will.*

Advanced dementia: a late severe stage of dementia.

Aggregate: in this book, refers to clumps of brain proteins (as well as the process of clumping), often toxic to brain cells around them. Microscopic protein aggregates are found in most neurodegenerative causes of dementia.

Aggression: a severe form of agitation with shouting or even physically aggressive behavior such as punching or kicking.

Agitation: heightened stress response expressed by the person with dementia, often accompanying delusions.

Allele: variations of a gene; some genes have many allelic variations, and some have only a handful.

Alzheimer's disease: the most common form of dementia in the world, mostly presenting as a progressive amnestic disorder with aging, but can also present with language, executive, visuospatial, physical, and behavioral symptoms. Alzheimer's disease clinical presentations often reflect the brain regions that are first or most affected. Its unifying microscopic hallmarks including clumped aggregates of brain proteins tau and amyloid.

Americans with Disabilities Act: a law precluding discrimination against a person for any disorder, including cognitive impairment.

Amnesia: forgetting.

Amnestic: forgetful.

Amyloid: also known as beta-amyloid or amyloid-beta; a protein implicated in Alzheimer's disease and several other forms of dementia. In such cases it is found in clumped aggregates around brain cells and is thought to be toxic or alternatively a marker of a toxic process. The presence or absence of brain amyloid can be determined by amyloid-PET imaging, lumbar puncture, and likely blood tests.

Amyloid-PET: a special type of positron emission tomography (PET) scan that can detect the presence or absence of amyloid in the brain to help determine the cause of dementia.

Amyloid-related imaging abnormalities (ARIA): the most common and serious side effect of intravenous anti-amyloid immunotherapies. ARIA include areas of brain swelling and bleeding, often only detected on MRI brain imaging.

Amyotrophic lateral sclerosis (ALS): a progressive neurodegenerative disorder, often rapidly progressive over months to years, with primary hallmarks of muscle weakness. It often leads to loss of swallowing and breathing. Also known as Lou Gehrig's disease (in the United States) or Charcot's disease (internationally).

Anhedonia: a lack of pleasure leading to loss of inertia or initiative; closely related to apathy.

Anticoagulant: a type of medication that acts by slowing the normal blood-clotting process. Often used to prevent strokes or other blood clots. Anticoagulant medications may be stopped in advance of some procedures such as a lumbar puncture.

Antipsychotics: a group of medications that can treat psychotic behavior in adults or aggressive and disruptive behaviors in dementia.

Aorta: the main artery exiting the heart and distributing blood throughout the body.

Apathy: loss of interest in doing things; closely related to anhedonia.

Aphasia: the inability to express or understand language.

Apolipoprotein E (APOE): a long-recognized risk gene for heart disease and Alzheimer's disease. Having one or two copies of the e4 variation increases the risk of Alzheimer's disease in some, but not all, people. The presence of APOE may be relevant to decisions about some medications used to treat Alzheimer's disease.

Arachnoid granulations: small structures at the top of the brain that reabsorb cerebrospinal fluid back into the bloodstream.

Arteriole: small branched arteries that carry oxygen-rich blood.

Artery: most often refers to a blood vessel that carries oxygen-rich blood throughout the body, including to the brain.

Artificial nutrition and hydration: food and water given by tubes inserted into either a vein in the arm or the stomach that usually sustain life but may not necessarily provide a high quality of life.

Aspiration pneumonia: a lung infection caused by accidentally inhaling food or saliva, often associated with advanced dementia.

Assisted living: residential facility that falls between independent living and a nursing home; provides a moderate amount of supervision and services and thus is usually a good fit for someone with mild to moderate dementia.

Astrocytes: brain cells that perform a complex array of functions, including physical and nutritional support.

Astrocytoma: a form of brain cancer primarily composed of abnormal astrocytes.

Atrial fibrillation: an irregular heart rhythm associated with clots developing in the heart. These clots can travel through the arteries to other regions of the body and cause blockages. In the brain these blockages cause strokes.

Atrophy: shrinkage of body tissue or an organ; in dementia, it refers to shrinkage of the brain and is associated with cognitive aging.

Attention: a cognitive skill of focusing or attending to one or more things.

Autonomic nervous system: responsible for the "fight or flight" reaction but also responsible for control and modulation of blood pressure and heart rate, body temperature, urination, bowel movements, and sexual functions.

Autopsy: a pathologic study of the body after death. A brain autopsy is the only way to definitively diagnose most forms of dementia.

Autosomal dominant: a genetic inheritance pattern in which half of people from one generation to the next appear to get a certain disease because one of two chromosomal variants is passed on.

Axons: long connections allowing communication from one neuron to the next.

B$_{12}$: also known as cobalamin or cyanocobalamin; low levels of vitamin B$_{12}$ can cause a range of neurologic symptoms, including cognitive impairment.

Basal ganglia: deep brain structures involved in facilitating movement and implicated in Parkinson's disease and other movement disorders.

Basic activities of daily living (BADLs): essential daily functions, such as personal hygiene (grooming and bathing), walking, eating, bathroom routines, and getting dressed.

Behavior: an observable and definable noncognitive function of the brain.

Behavioral and psychological symptoms of dementia (BPSD): a set of changes in mood, behavior, or sleep that accompany dementia. Behavioral and psychological symptoms of dementia can be a source of significant dementia-associated disability and caregiver stress. Also known as neuropsychiatric symptoms (NPS).

Behavioral neurologist: a specially trained neurologist (physician) with expertise in disorders of behavior and cognition, most often dementia.

Behavioral-variant frontotemporal dementia (FTD): a form of frontotemporal dementia that primarily causes changes in personality.

Benzodiazepines: a group of antianxiety medications for adults that are also used to help control aggression, insomnia, and disruptive behaviors in dementia.

Biomarker: a finding from an objective test usually associated with brain imaging, blood, or cerebrospinal fluid that, when present, is indicative of a disease such as dementia.

Biopsy: a specimen from the body taken surgically and sent for pathological review.

Bipolar disorder: a group of common psychiatric disorders involving dramatic and often sustained swings or variations in mood ranging from depression to hyperactivity. Onset is usually in late adolescence into young adulthood. Also known as bipolar affective disorder or bipolar disease.

Blood–brain barrier: the tight barrier between the capillaries and the brain that limits toxins, germs, and even medications from entering the brain.

Blood clot: a stoppage of blood flow in either the arteries (which carry oxygenated blood from the lungs to the body) or the veins (which carry deoxygenated blood from the periphery to the heart and back to the lungs).

Blood vessel: an artery or vein carrying blood in the body.

Bovine spongiform encephalopathy: a now rare if not eradicated form of prion disease seen in cows.

BPSD: see *behavioral and psychological symptoms of dementia.*

Brainstem: the lower part or back part of the brain, responsible for awareness, facial movements and feeling, and connecting the brain to the spinal cord.

CADASIL (cerebral autosomal dominant arteriopathy with subcortical infarcts and leukoencephalopathy): a genetic cause of subcortical white matter strokes and cognitive impairment.

Capillary: the smallest vessel in the brain; carries nutrients and oxygen to brain tissue.

Caregiver: someone who is engaged in the coordination and/or delivery of care to another person, such as someone contending with a dementia diagnosis. Caregivers can be professionals or friends/family members.

Care partner: someone who is engaged in facilitating and often advocating for care in the earliest stages of cognitive changes when the affected person is fully capable of directing others.

Carotid arteries: a pair of arteries in the front of the neck that supply blood to the brain.

Central nervous system: the brain and spinal cord.

Cerebellum: the back area of the brain, largely responsible for coordination and balance.

Cerebral amyloid angiopathy (CAA): a brain blood vessel disease causing strokes that is strongly associated with Alzheimer's disease.

Cerebrospinal fluid (CSF): a clear, colorless, naturally occurring fluid created by and surrounding the brain.

Cerebrum or cerebral cortex: area of the brain with the principal areas responsible for the brain's higher-order abilities.

Charles Bonnet syndrome: a normal brain phenomenon in which hallucinated images are created by the brain when primary vision is failing. This may be most apparent in low-lit environments.

Cholinesterase inhibitors: medications that slow the breakdown of the neurotransmitter acetylcholine. In dementia, these medications are used to treat Alzheimer's disease, Lewy body dementia, and vascular dementia.

Choroid plexus: small structures deep in the brain that make cerebrospinal fluid.

Chronic traumatic encephalopathy (CTE): the neuropathological changes seen in persons with the clinical traumatic encephalopathy syndrome (TES). CTE and TES are thought to follow years of exposure to chronic low-impact hits to the head as are seen in contact sports such as football and boxing.

Cognition: thinking, memory, perception, or language function of the brain.

Cognitive: term describing a thinking, memory, perception, or language function of the brain.

Cognitive impairment: a relative deficit in thinking and memory abilities. Primary cognitive domains that may be impaired include memory, language, executive, and visuospatial function.

Cognitive reserve: the concept that people who have experienced a more cognitively rich lifestyle across their lifespan, beginning with a longer and richer educational history and continuing into professional attainment/job complexity as well as cognitive leisure experiences across a lifetime, are less likely to experience dementia until later in life or until more severe brain disease is apparent.

Comfort feeding: a way to deliver nutrition once someone is unable to eat in the terminal stage of dementia. Small quantities of food are hand fed to the patient as long as obvious choking does not follow. Comfort feeding helps address the potentially distressing perception that no food or nutrition is being given.

Comprehensive lifestyle decisions: diet, exercise, socialization, and cognitive stimulation advised as a nonpharmacologic strategy to help with dementia.

Computed tomography scan: a high-resolution x-ray image of the brain; also called CT or CAT scan.

Corticobasal degeneration: a form of corticobasal syndrome specifically caused by the microscopic changes of frontotemporal dementia.

Corticobasal syndrome: a type of dementia, either Alzheimer's disease or frontotemporal dementia, with hallmarks of one-sided physical motor symptoms along with language and visuospatial dysfunction.

Crystallized knowledge: someone's personal, established knowledge learned through formal education and autobiographical experiences.

CSF: see *cerebrospinal fluid.*

CT scan: see *computed tomography scan.*

DaT scan: see *dopamine transporter (DaT) scan.*

Day programs: community-based social programs offering cognitive enrichment for seniors, often lasting several hours each time; also known as geriatric social day programs.

Decisional capacity: the ability to weigh information and make decisions based on medical facts.

Decubitus ulcer: a skin wound that begins within minutes to hours of not moving. When severe, decubitus ulcers can be complicated by infections that can become serious and overwhelming if not recognized quickly. Also known as a bedsore or pressure ulcer.

Delirium: a medical condition characterized by confusion or fatigue that is out of character for the person with dementia, often accompanied by fluctuations in cognitive function and psychotic features, including hallucinations. It usually develops over the course of hours or days and is often a sign of a serious medical problem such as a medication side effect, infection, or stroke.

Delusions: fixed false beliefs.

Dementia: an umbrella term given to a group of disorders that collectively cause someone to have difficulty in thinking, speaking, remembering, or behaving in the way that they did during their normal adult life.

Dementia pugilistica: an older term for traumatic encephalopathy syndrome.

Dementia with Lewy bodies: the second most common cause of progressive neurodegenerative dementia, primarily due to Lewy bodies in the brain. Key features include cognitive impairment, fluctuations, visual hallucinations, and rapid-eye-movement (REM) sleep behavior disorder, which precedes or occurs at the same time as parkinsonism. It is one of several Lewy body dementias.

Depression: a common mental health disorder with features of sadness or the blues.

Diabetes: a non-neurologic disorder of sugar intolerance that is associated with increased risk of heart attacks, stroke, kidney failure, and dementia.

Disease-modifying therapies: medications that target underlying causes and biological changes of disease rather than just symptoms of disease.

DNA: deoxyribonucleic acid, the human genetic code.

Dopamine transporter (DaT) scan: a form of single-photon computed tomography that focuses on the dopamine transporter and helps in differentiating causes of parkinsonism.

Dream enactment: acting out dreams, often part of dementia with Lewy bodies.

Dysarthria: problems articulating speech.

Dysphagia: problems with swallowing.

Early-onset dementia: defined as dementia beginning by age 60.

EEG: see *electroencephalogram.*

Electroencephalogram (EEG): brainwave test used to diagnose seizures.

Ependyma: inner layer or lining around the brain ventricles.

Ependymal cells: cells that make up the ependyma

Epilepsy: a neurologic disease with multiple recurring seizures.

Executive dysfunction: cognitive impairment with hallmarks of difficulty focusing and learning multiple pieces of information and problems with planning or following a sequence.

Executive skills: complex cognitive abilities involving multitasking, planning, and responding to changing information.

Executor of an estate: a person who carries out the wishes conveyed in a will.

FAST: see *Functional Assessment Staging.*

Fatal familial insomnia: a form of Creutzfeldt–Jakob disease with prominent features of insomnia.

FDG-PET: a form of PET scan that highlights regions of relative brain function, using a small infusion of a radioactive tracer linked to glucose or sugar.

Fluctuations: variability in cognition or motor features from day to day or within a day, often seen in dementia with Lewy bodies.

Fluorodeoxyglucose (FDG): a radiolabeled form of glucose, or sugar, used in PET imaging; see *FDG-PET.*

Frontal-executive: the term emphasizing the executive skills generated by the frontal lobes. The term can also refer to the clinically apparent presentation of dementia, such as the frontal-executive form of Alzheimer's disease, in which executive dysfunction is the most apparent initial problem.

Frontal lobe (frontal cortex): front area of the brain responsible for complex thoughts, planning, and personality, among other functions.

Frontotemporal dementia (FTD): a form of dementia involving either prominent behavioral or language changes.

Frontotemporal lobar degeneration (FTLD): a group of neurodegenerative brain diseases including frontotemporal dementia, progressive supranuclear palsy, and corticobasal degeneration. This umbrella term is most often found in technical or research settings and is used to capture several less common forms of dementia with overlapping symptoms, microscopic changes, and genetic causes, but it is not often used in clinical practice.

Functional Assessment Staging (FAST): a screening tool to determine dementia stage, often used in planning for hospice enrollment.

Functional neuroimaging: a brain imaging technique highlighting brain function over brain structure. Positron emission tomography (PET) is an example.

Gait: the manner in which someone walks; often formally assessed during physician visits.

Gene: a microscopic code that leads to a normal human bodily function but can also cause a disease.

General medical examination: the part of the medical examination not focused on neurologic signs.

Gene therapy: treatments focused on altering or introducing a change in the genetic code.

Genetic counselor: a nonphysician specialist whose role is to explain and anticipate complex personal and family issues around testing, anticipating, and understanding information related to genetic testing.

Geriatrician: a general medical doctor specially trained in treating aging or geriatric patients.

Gerstmann–Sträussler–Scheinker syndrome: a form of Creutzfeldt–Jakob disease with prominent ataxia and parkinsonism.

Glia: a broad group of cells that includes oligodendrocytes, astrocytes, ependymal cells, and microglia, among others.

Glioblastoma or glioblastoma multiforme (GBM): a primary and aggressive brain tumor that can present with or cause dementia if it involves brain structures important for cognitive abilities.

Glucose: a form of sugar used as an energy source in most cells of the body. Glucose is also used in brain imaging; see *FDG-PET*.

Glutamate: a toxic neurotransmitter in the brain.

Gray matter: the outer part of the brain where most of the neurons are.

Health care agent: a person who is designated legally through a health care proxy to make health decisions on behalf of someone who cannot make decisions for themselves. In the absence of a proxy, a health care surrogate may become the health care agent.

Health care proxy: a document legally designating a health care agent to make health decisions when someone is unable to do so for themselves. In common use, health care proxy is used interchangeably in describing the person who is the health care agent.

Health care surrogate: in the absence of a health care proxy, a legal next of kin, close friend, or appointed guardian who is designated as the health care agent.

Heidenhain variant of Creutzfeldt–Jakob disease: a form of Creutzfeldt–Jakob disease with prominent visuospatial symptoms.

Hemisphere: a half of the brain.

Hemorrhage: a bleed.

Hemorrhagic stroke: a type of stroke due to a break in a blood vessel with bleeding.

Hippocampus: a key area of the brain responsible for short-term memory that is implicated in Alzheimer's disease.

HIV: see *human immunodeficiency virus*.

Hospice: a system allowing for supportive and palliative care when life expectancy is less than 6 months.

Human immunodeficiency virus (HIV): a viral infection that causes immune suppression and if untreated can lead to a series of life-threatening secondary or opportunistic infections also known as acquired immune deficiency syndrome (AIDS).

Hydrocephalus: an excessive amount of cerebrospinal fluid within the brain. Two types of hydrocephalus exist, communicating and non-communicating, referring to whether or not there is a blockage in how the cerebrospinal fluid naturally flows through channels deep within the brain.

Hypertension: high blood pressure, a common stroke risk factor that is often manageable with medications and home monitoring.

IADLs: see *instrumental activities of daily living.*

Illusion: in this book, a misinterpretation of an image or object for something else; often a part of dementia with Lewy bodies

Inclusion body: a collection or clumping of protein often found in neurodegenerative disease, either in the cell body or nucleus.

Incontinence: typically refers to the inability to hold urine or stool. May also refer to emotions, such as when someone is unable to hold in laughter or crying, often at inappropriate times.

Independent living: a level of geriatric care allowing some degree of freedom and minimal assistance or supervision.

Inherited disorder: a disease passed down from one generation to the next in some families due to a shared gene.

Instrumental activities of daily living (IADLs): a host of things that one must be able to accomplish independently as an adult to continue to thrive.

Interventional studies: research in which people with a disease are assigned a treatment and outcomes are observed.

In vitro fertilization (IVF): a process by which an egg is fertilized outside the body. Some families carrying genes that cause dementia or other diseases may use IVF to ensure that the gene stops getting passed to the next generation of family members.

Ischemic stroke: a stroke caused by a blockage of blood flow in the brain.

Late-onset dementia: dementia that begins at age 61 years or later.

Leukodystrophies: diseases of the white matter in the brain and spinal cord.

Lewy body: a microscopic aggregated round inclusion of α-synuclein located in brain neurons.

Lewy body dementias: group of dementias including Parkinson's disease dementia, dementia with Lewy bodies, and the Lewy body variant of Alzheimer's disease.

Lewy body disease: a group of brain diseases that includes Parkinson's disease, Parkinson's disease dementia, dementia with Lewy bodies, and the Lewy body variant of Alzheimer's disease, all of which involve Lewy body microscopic changes. These diseases have overlapping features of dementia with parkinsonism, memory loss, prominent sleep behavioral problems, and visual hallucinations.

Lewy body variant of Alzheimer's disease: Variant of Alzheimer's disease in which microscopic Lewy body changes occur in the brain. It affects about one-third of all people with Alzheimer's disease. When both changes are present, people will mostly have features of Alzheimer's disease, including memory loss and brain atrophy on MRI, but also have some of the behavioral features of dementia with Lewy bodies, including visual hallucinations, fluctuations, and REM sleep behavior disorder.

Lidocaine: a common local anesthetic medication that is used to numb skin and underlying tissue during some procedures, including a lumbar puncture (spinal tap).

Living will: a document that details a person's wishes about how they wish to receive medical care during severe life-threatening illness or in advancing stages of dementia; also known as an advance directive.

Logopenia: an abnormal amount of word-finding difficulty that may occur in dementia or stroke.

Logopenic primary progressive aphasia: a form of dementia with prominent aphasia, particularly logopenia.

Long-term care insurance policy: a voluntary policy offered by insurance companies that defrays the cost of some of the more expensive services associated with dementia care, including personnel (home health aides), respite, and nursing home support.

Lou Gehrig's disease: an American term used for amyotrophic lateral sclerosis. Lou Gehrig was a famous baseball player whose career was cut short by the disease

Lumbar puncture: a medical procedure in which cerebrospinal fluid is collected for diagnostic and analytic purposes; also known as a spinal tap.

Magnetic gait: a walking abnormality seen in normal pressure hydrocephalus in which the feet appear to be stuck to the floor.

Magnetic resonance imaging (MRI): a high-resolution nonradiating image of the brain generated using pulsating magnets.

Major neurocognitive disorder: a recently coined synonym for dementia; likely to be used only in the medical profession.

MCI: see *mild cognitive impairment.*

Mechanical ventilation: an artificial means or device used to support breathing.

Memory: the ability to recall verbal or nonverbal information. Memory can refer to working memory (remembering in the moment), short-term memory (memory from minutes to hours ago), long-term memory (information held from events long ago), declarative memory (information about events or people), and procedural memory (memory for tasks, often involving sequences of smaller tasks).

Meningioma: the most common tumor within the head; meningiomas are often benign but can cause neurologic problems, including cognitive impairment or behavioral changes, if they become large enough to compress structures important to those functions.

Metabolic disorders: a broad term used to describe a host of medical problems that may alter the body and brain chemistry and cause or worsen cognitive problems. Examples include infections, kidney or liver failure, and dehydration.

Microglia: the brain's immune system cells, which able to fight infection but also responsible for generating inflammatory changes.

Microscopic: something very small, usually referring to a body tissue, seen only under a microscope.

Microvascular: small blood vessels. In this book, the term is used to describe diseases and brain imaging findings suggesting small strokes.

Mild cognitive impairment (MCI): a state, often transitional and occurring before people develop dementia, in which objective and subjective indicators of cognitive impairment are noted but do not have functional impact on instrumental activities of daily living.

Minor neurocognitive disorder: a recently coined synonym for mild cognitive impairment, likely to be used only in the medical profession.

Monogenetic: associated with a single gene.

Mood: a perceived state of well-being. Abnormal moods include depression and anxiety.

Motor neuron disease (MND): see *amyotrophic lateral sclerosis.*

Motor neurons: nerve cells in the spinal cord that move the arms, legs, and trunk. In this book, they become affected in amyotrophic lateral sclerosis.

MRI: see *magnetic resonance imaging.*

Multiple sclerosis (MS): a disease of the central nervous system involving inflammatory demyelinating lesions of the white matter. Patients with MS experience focal neurologic symptoms in discrete episodes over time, often seemingly unrelated to one another. MS is a relatively common neurologic disease, with onset most often in young adult women; diagnosis is usually made by a combination of history, imaging, and cerebrospinal fluid analysis.

Myelin: a substance created by cells in the nervous system that coats the long axons and white matter fibers that connect nerve cells. When myelin is damaged, electrical signals are interrupted in the nervous system.

Neologism: a nonsensical word or sound.

Nervous system: the set of nerves and their connections in the body.

Neural networks: circuits of nerve cells within the brain.

Neurodegeneration: the process in which a single group of cells begin to become sick, wither, and die either simultaneously or in some sequence that is difficult to determine.

Neurologic examination: the part of a doctor's physical examination that focuses on the neurologic system.

Neurologist: a doctor specializing in diseases of the nervous system, including dementia.

Neuron: a nerve cell that communicates with other nerve cells by electrical signals.

Neuropathologically: referring to something seen or identified through microscopic review of nervous system tissue.

Neuropathology: neurologic changes seen on gross inspection of a part of the nervous system or under a microscope.

Neuropsychiatric symptoms (NPS): another term for behavioral and psychological symptoms of dementia.

Neuropsychiatrist: a neurologist or psychiatrist with special training focused on cognitive and behavioral disorders.

Neuropsychological testing: a noninvasive test or set of tests that can identify specific domains of cognitive abilities or difficulties and is particularly useful at identifying whether cognitive changes are those that may be expected to accompany age or not based on normal findings known to occur in others with similar backgrounds, as well as providing an estimate of when changes may be meaningful for the person being tested.

Neuropsychologist: a (nonphysician) psychologist who provides neuropsychological testing and interpretation and, often, counseling.

Neurotransmitter: a chemical signal sent between two nerve cells.

Neurovascular unit: the coupling of the blood vessel to a neuron and its surrounding cells and microenvironment.

N-methyl-D-aspartate (NMDA): a type of brain receptor that triggers the release of a toxic neurotransmitter called glutamate.

Nonamnestic: a form of cognitive impairment in which memory is rather normal or of particular strength relative to other cognitive deficiencies. A person with primary language problems in dementia may be described as having non-amnestic cognitive impairment.

Normal pressure hydrocephalus: a form of communicating hydrocephalus presenting with a triad of dementia, magnetic gait, and urinary incontinence.

Nuclear medicine: a medical specialty in which radioactive medications are used for diagnostic and treatment purposes. In the field of dementia, nuclear medicine relates to special brain imaging (see Appendix A).

Nursing home: technically an inpatient facility for long-term residents who do not have acute care needs; also known as residential care, memory care, or subacute nursing facility.

Observational studies: research that does not involve an intervention or treatment but instead tracks the natural history of a group of people.

Obstructive sleep apnea: a disorder of breathing during sleep in which the upper airway is obstructed. Symptoms include snoring and brief periods of no breathing during sleep, often followed by deep breaths. Phases of normal sleep are disrupted, and this disruption can lead to daytime fatigue, reduced daytime vigilance, and impaired executive abilities.

Occipital lobe (occipital cortex): the area of the brain responsible for vision.

Oligodendrocytes: the cells in the brain that make myelin in the white matter.

Oligodendroglioma: a form of brain cancer primarily composed of cells that create brain myelin.

Onset: in this text, refers to the age at which dementia begins. This is in contrast to stage, which refers to the severity or phase of disease. See *early-onset dementia* and *late-onset dementia*.

Orthostatic hypotension: a drop in blood pressure and a failure of the autonomic system to respond to changes in body position, such as transitions from lying down or sitting to a standing position. This often accompanies dementia with Lewy bodies and Parkinson's disease.

Paraphasias: word errors that may be nearly correct in thought or sound.

Parietal lobe (parietal cortex): brain region responsible for sensory, perceptual, and information integration.

Parkinsonian: having motor features of parkinsonism.

Parkinsonism: stiffness, slowness, rigidity, and/or tremor. These are symptoms of Parkinson's disease and can be seen in a broad range of neurodegenerative dementias as well as after stroke.

Parkinson's disease: a progressive neurodegenerative disease with features of stiffness, slowness, rigidity, and/or tremor, often beginning with a tremor that occurs only at rest and in one hand.

Pathophysiology: the underlying biochemical and microscopic changes of a disease, often associated with an apparent cause.

Penetrance: the likelihood that a person who has a gene associated with a particular disease, such as dementia, will develop the disease.

Peripheral nervous system: the nervous system of the body that includes (a) the motor nerves that exit the spinal cord and brainstem, causing stimulation and movement of muscles in the body, and (b) the sensory nerves carrying information from the skin and body back to the spinal cord and brainstem.

PET scan: see *positron emission tomography scan.*

Phase 1 studies: the earliest stage of interventional studies; in this phase, the safety of a new medication is explored in up to several dozen healthy persons and a handful of persons with a disease.

Phase 2 studies: interventional studies, typically of new medications, that enroll several hundred people and are principally focused on safety but may begin to show possible efficacy.

Phase 3 studies: interventional studies of drugs that have already been shown to be safe in phase 2 but are now being studied in a few thousand people with the intent of demonstrating efficacy.

Phlebotomy: the process of drawing blood, such as from a vein in the arm.

Physiatrist: a doctor specializing in physical medicine and rehabilitation. In dementia, a physiatrist may help with supporting or recovering mobility.

Pick's disease: an older term previously used to describe frontotemporal dementia. Pick body is a term still in use that describes specific microscopic changes seen in brain cells of some people with frontotemporal dementia.

Placebo: the inactive or inert arm of an interventional study. Whether a participant is receiving a placebo or the active drug is usually not known to either the participant or the treating physician until later in the study. Some call a placebo a "sugar pill," but this term is not accurate nor relevant to those receiving infusions.

Plasma: a fluid phase of the blood that contains circulating proteins. New tests can detect amyloid and tau in the blood and may have an increasing role in diagnosing Alzheimer's disease and other dementias.

POLST: a portable medical order that informs code status and other advance directives.

Polysomnogram: an overnight sleep study used to diagnose breathing or neurologic problems causing disrupted sleep, particularly sleep apnea and REM-sleep behavior disorders.

Positron emission tomography (PET) scan: a nuclear medicine scan used to determine a cause of dementia. See *FDG-PET* and *amyloid-PET*.

Posterior cortical atrophy: focal atrophy or shrinkage of the rear parts of the brain. Most often, posterior cortical atrophy is associated with complex visuospatial symptoms with microscopic evidence of Alzheimer's disease. Early symptoms may include difficulty reading without evidence of problems in the eye.

Power of attorney: a legal document designating another person to make financial decisions in your absence. A durable power of attorney also allows that person to make financial decisions if you become cognitively impaired and cannot make decisions for yourself. Both forms of power of attorney end upon death.

PPA: see *primary progressive aphasia*.

Primary progressive aphasia (PPA): a set of disorders causing dementia by gradually impairing language.

Prion: a brain protein implicated in Creutzfeldt–Jakob disease.

Processing speed: the pace or speed with which the brain considers and acts in response to a stimulus. Can be objectively determined by some timed tasks on neuropsychological testing.

Progenitor cell: an early cell type specific to a tissue or organ that can occur anywhere in the body.

Progressive nonfluent aphasia: a primary progressive aphasia form of frontotemporal dementia with halting speech as its main hallmark.

Progressive supranuclear palsy (PSP): part of the frontotemporal dementia spectrum of disorders; the best-recognized form of progressive supranuclear palsy has features of parkinsonism, poor balance including falling backward, and impaired vertical eye movements. The microscopic changes of progressive supranuclear palsy are now found in a range of other clinical presentations, including cognitive impairment or, more typically, Parkinson's disease.

Protein aggregation: the process of clumping of brain proteins. See *aggregate*.

Proteins: basic chemical building blocks found throughout the body and nature, present in all living things.

Proxy: in this book, refers to a person serving in a position to make medical decisions on behalf of another. Technically, a health care proxy is the document that designates a health care agent, but the terms are used interchangeably in common language to describe the agent or person.

Pseudobulbar affect: a change seen in progressive supranuclear palsy, after stroke, or in some people with amyotrophic lateral sclerosis, with hallmarks of uncontrollable laughter or crying.

Psychiatrist: a physician whose practice focuses on diagnosing and treating disorders of mood and behavior.

Psychological: a term reflecting objectively defined symptoms of mood or behavior.

Psychologist: a nonphysician provider, often referred to as a therapist, whose practice focuses on treating disorders of mood or behavior through various forms of nonpharmacologic treatment; often works in conjunction with a psychiatrist.

Radioloabel: a "tag" or linked chemical connection made between a biological substance and a radioactive particle. When a radiolabeled compound is injected or otherwise placed into the body, a scanning machine can detect where the biological substance is active or inactive in the body.

Rapid eye movement (REM): a period of sleep in which the brain is very active; the eyes rapidly move about while the limbs remain still. Dreaming often occurs during this period of sleep.

Rapid eye movement (REM) sleep behavior disorder: a set of abnormal behaviors that occur during REM sleep that may include dream enactment (acting out dreams), somniloquy (sleeptalking), and, less often, somnambulism (sleepwalking). These often precede or are profound in those with dementia with Lewy bodies or Parkinson's disease dementia.

Reorienting strategies: a term describing a collective technique to support a person with dementia by nonpharmacologic means, often to break a cycle of forgetfulness, de-escalate emerging agitation, or prevent neuropsychiatric problems altogether. Approaches include changing the environment to remove potentially stressful triggers, maintaining a supportive tone, and using diversions and distractions.

Sandwich generation: a person responsible for providing care for both the previous and next generation of family members (i.e., parents and children).

Schizophrenia: a complex but common psychiatric disorder of disorganized thought and psychosis that usually begins in adolescence through early adulthood.

Seizure: a single event of excessive electrical brain activity that can cause a range of changes such as shaking in parts of the body or just changes in awareness. Someone who experiences many seizures over time is said to have epilepsy.

Semantic dementia: a primary progressive aphasia form of frontotemporal dementia causing loss of knowledge of information and the context of words.

Semantics: the meanings of words or characteristics of objects, such as their use or context.

Sensed presence: a complex visual symptom sometimes seen in dementia with Lewy bodies in which a person thinks there is an object, animal, or person just outside their field of vision or around a corner of a room from them.

Side effects: unintended effects of a drug or other therapy.

Signs: objective or observed findings on medical and neurologic examinations. In contrast, *symptoms* are problems reported as perceived by a person or their care partner.

Single-photon-emission computed tomography (SPECT): a means of determining brain metabolism; provides similar information to positron emission tomography.

Sleep apnea: a disorder when breathing stops during sleep. See *obstructive sleep apnea.*

Somnambulism: sleepwalking.

Somniloquy: sleeptalking.

SPECT: see *single-photon-emission computed tomography.*

Spinal cord: a network of nerve fibers transmitting signals from the brain to the limbs and torso and vice versa.

Spinal drain: an extended form of a lumbar puncture in which a small plastic catheter is placed into the spinal canal and left to drain fluid for hours to days and monitor for clinical response. In dementia, this is a technique used to diagnose normal pressure hydrocephalus when a spinal tap is not fully informative. In contrast to a lumbar puncture, a spinal drain requires an inpatient hospital stay.

Spinal tap: see *lumbar puncture.*

Stage: in this text, refers to the phase or severity of dementia. The early stage involves mild symptoms, and the late stage refers to end phases of disease. Stage is in contrast to *onset*, which refers to the age at which dementia first becomes symptomatic.

Stem cell: an early cell type that can form into any cell in the body.

Strategic single cerebral infarct dementia: a single large stroke that may cause dementia.

Stroke: a sudden event in the brain when a blood supply is cut off by a blockage (ischemic stroke) or when a blood vessel ruptures (hemorrhagic stroke).

Structural causes of dementia: a group of diseases including masses or fluid retention that compress or invade the brain and cause cognitive impairment.

Subacute nursing facility: a center providing care usually for recently hospitalized patients who are only able to engage in a minimal amount of rehabilitative services. Patients admitted to these centers may stay for an extended period of time.

Subcortical: in the deep part of the brain, this is often how the white matter is referred to.

Subcortical white matter microvascular disease: a multiplicity of small white matter changes causing strokes.

Subdural hematoma: a posttraumatic collection of blood around the brain. When large or bilateral, subdural hematoma can cause cognitive impairment and other neurologic problems.

Sundowning: episodes of behavioral and psychological symptoms of dementia occurring late in the day.

Swallowing evaluation: a test performed by a speech and language pathologist to determine whether a patient is at risk for choking.

Symptoms: problems perceived, felt, or noticed by a person or others and reported to a doctor. In contrast, *signs* are findings objectively identified on examination.

Synuclein: a brain protein implicated in dementia with Lewy bodies, Parkinson's disease, and several other neurodegenerative brain diseases; also known as α-synuclein.

Syphilis: a sexually transmitted infectious disease; if untreated, it can cause a range of neurologic problems, including cognitive impairment and stroke.

Tangles: in this book, refers to clumped tau proteins, also known as *neurofibrillary tangles.*

Tau: a brain protein implicated in Alzheimer's disease, the frontotemporal dementias, and several other neurodegenerative brain diseases.

Tau-PET: a special form of positron emission tomography (PET) scan that can detect the presence or absence of tau in the brain to help determine the cause of dementia.

TDP-43: a brain protein implicated in frontotemporal dementia. Sometimes TDP-43 aggregates can present in brain regions implicated in Alzheimer's disease and cause similar symptoms.

Temporal lobe (temporal cortex): the part of the brain responsible for new memory and language.

Terminal decline: the final severe stage of dementia in which basic functions of mobility and cognition, as well as automatic abilities to chew and swallow, are lost, followed only by death.

Thrombectomy: physical retrieval and removal of a clot that has lodged in an artery; in this book, it refers to a time-sensitive stroke treatment.

Thyroid disease: a dysfunction of the thyroid gland. A low-functioning thyroid (hypothyroid) can cause signs and symptoms of dementia.

Thyroid gland: an endocrine organ located in the front of the neck that produces a hormone that regulates the level of function and energy use of nearly every other organ and cell in the body. A low-functioning thyroid can cause fatigue, constipation, a feeling of being cold, depression, and memory problems.

Trachea: the windpipe in the throat.

Traumatic encephalopathy syndrome (TES): the clinical syndrome associated with chronic traumatic encephalopathy, following years of exposure to multiple mild traumatic brain injuries as seen in some sports. Clinical features include cognitive impairment, mood and behavioral changes, and sometimes parkinsonism.

Tremor: a rhythmic shaking of a limb, head, jaw, trunk, or voice that may occur with rest, posture, or action. Tremor usually stops during sleep.

Trust: a legal document to establish directors responsible for financial management during a person's lifetime.

Urinary tract infection: an infection in the bladder, kidneys, their connections (ureters), or the tube through which urine passes (urethra).

Vascular dementia: dementia due to strokes, either single large strokes or many small strokes. These strokes can be ischemic or hemorrhagic.

Ventricles: large areas of the brain filled with cerebrospinal fluid.

Ventriculoperitoneal shunt: a long multi-section tube placed into the brain and tunneled beneath the skin, eventually ending in the abdomen. It is the most common surgical treatment for normal pressure hydrocephalus.

Verbal memory: memory for learning and remembering a story or a list of unrelated words.

Vertebral arteries: a pair of arteries in the back of the neck supplying blood to the brainstem and rear parts of the brain.

Visual hallucination: a visual perception seen only by the affected person. Visual hallucinations can be simple (colors, flashes) or complex (shapes, animals, people); in this book, visual hallucinations are most relevant to dementia with Lewy bodies.

Visuospatial: usually an adjective used with abilities or function; often refers to one's ability to determine one's relative position in the environment (e.g., navigational tasks such as driving, following directions, and determining distance).

Visuospatial impairment: the inability to correctly determine the relative position of oneself to the environment or the relative position of two objects to one another. Symptoms of visuospatial impairment include getting lost in or on the way to familiar places or having difficulty avoiding the furniture in a room.

Visuospatial memory: memory for remembering a planned path or series of intended directions.

Vitamin deficiency: a low level of an essential dietary micronutrient.

White matter: the myelin-rich parts of the central nervous system, which largely are areas with pathways for neurons sending electrical signals.

Will: a legal document that provides directions for the transfer of one's wealth after death.

Word salad: a set of nonsensical word-like sounds.

ABOUT THE *BRAIN & LIFE* AND THE AMERICAN ACADEMY OF NEUROLOGY

Brain & Life® is the only magazine and website focused on the intersection of brain health and neurologic disease. A print subscription to *Brain & Life* (six issues a year) is available for free to anyone residing in the United States. Visit *BrainandLife.org* to subscribe or read stories on brain science, brain health and wellness, and living well with neurologic disorders.

Brain & Life is an official publication of the American Academy of Neurology (AAN). Founded in 1948, the AAN represents more than 38,000 members who are neurologists and neuroscience professionals and is dedicated to promoting the highest quality patient-centered neurologic care. A neurologist is a doctor with specialized training in diagnosing, treating, and managing disorders of the brain and nervous system such as Alzheimer's disease, stroke, migraine, multiple sclerosis, concussion, Parkinson's disease, and epilepsy. For more information about the American Academy of Neurology, visit *AAN.com*.

INDEX

For the benefit of digital users, indexed terms that span two pages (e.g., 52–53) may, on occasion, appear on only one of those pages.

Tables and figures are indicated by *t* and *f* following the page number.